GET THROUGH MEDICAL SCHOOL

GET THROUGH MEDICAL SCHOOL: 1000 SBAs/BOFs AND EMQs

By

Una Coales
MD FRCS FRCS (Oto) DRCOG DFFP
General Practice Registrar
London Deanery
London, UK

Seema Khan
MBBS
Graduate of Guy's,
King's and St Thomas'
School of Medicine

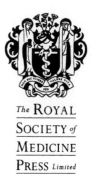

The ROYAL
SOCIETY of
MEDICINE
PRESS Limited

© 2003 Royal Society of Medicine Press Ltd
Reprinted 2004

1 Wimpole Street, London W1G 0AE
207 Westminster Road, Lake Forest IL 60045 USA
www.rsmpress.co.uk

British Library Cataloguing in Publication Data
A catalogue record for this book is available from the British Library

ISBN: 1–85315–546–2

Typeset by Phoenix Photosetting, Chatham, Kent

Printed in Great Britain by Bell and Bain Ltd., Glasgow

Contents

Preface

Medical schools in the UK are changing the format of examinations and adopting the popular style of single best answers (SBAs)/best of fives (BOFs) and extended matching questions (EMQs). Currently there are no books on the market aimed at medical students that address this new format. This book presents 1000 clinically relevant SBAs/BOFs and EMQs and covers the core curriculum of medicine, surgery, psychiatry, obstetrics and gynaecology and paediatrics. The emphasis in each subject is proportionate to that represented in medical school finals, with more emphasis placed on medicine and surgery. The questions also encompass clinical scenarios likely to be encountered as a house officer. This is a valuable book not only for passing medical school examinations but also for preparing you to manage patients as a house officer or at the senior house officer grade.

This book is a collaboration by both a junior doctor who has recently passed the new format of medical school finals and by a doctor with several years of hospital experience at the SHO and registrar levels.

We would like to thank Dr Phil Timms, Senior Lecturer in Community Psychiatry, United Medical and Dental Schools, St Thomas' Hospital for his editorial input for the questions on psychiatry.

Una Coales
Seema Khan

October, 2002

Recommended Texts and References

Medicine

The Editorial Board (2001) *Advanced Life Support Course Provider Manual*. Resuscitation Council (UK), London.

Braunwald E. *et al.* (2001) *Harrison's Principles of Internal Medicine*, 15th edn. McGraw-Hill, New York.

Longmore J.M. *et al.* (2001) *Oxford Handbook of Clinical Medicine*, 5th edn. Oxford University Press, Oxford.

Kumar P.J. *et al.* (2002) *Clinical Medicine*, 5th edn. W.B. Saunders, London.

Royal Pharmaceutical Society of Great Britain (2001) *British National Formulary*. British Medical Association, London.

Rubenstein D. *et al.* (2002) *Lecture Notes on Clinical Medicine*, 6th edn. Blackwell Science Publications, Oxford.

Surgery

Ellis H. (2002*) Lecture Notes on General Surgery*, 10th edn. Blackwell Science, Oxford.

Harken A.H. & Moore E. (2000) *Surgical Secrets*, 4th edn. Hanley & Belfus, Philadephia.

Lattimer C.R. *et al.* (1996) *Key Topics in General Surgery*, 1st edn. BIOS Scientific Publishers, Oxford.

McLatchie G.R. (2001) *Oxford Handbook of Clinical Surgery*, 2nd edn. Oxford University Press, Oxford.

Roland N.J. *et al.* (1995) *Key Topics in Otolaryngology*, 1st edn. BIOS Scientific Publishers, Oxford.

Solomon L. *et al.* (2001) *Apley's System of Orthopaedics and Fractures*, 8th edn. Arnold, London.

Unwin A. *et al.* (1995) *Emergency Orthopaedics and Trauma*, 1st edn. Butterworth-Heinemann, Oxford.

Psychiatry

American Psychiatric Association (2000) *Diagnostic and Statistic Manual of Mental Disorders*, 4th edn. American Psychiatric Association, Washington D.C.

Davies T. *et al.* (1998) *ABC of Mental Health*, 1st edn. BMJ Books, London.

Tomb, D.A. (1999) *Psychiatry*, 6th edn. Lippincott, Williams and Wilkins, Baltimore.

Obstetrics and gynaecology

Chamberlain G. & Hamilton-Fairly D. (1999) *Lecture Notes on Obstetrics & Gynaecology*. Blackwell Science, Oxford.

Collier J.A.B. *et al.* (1999) *Oxford Handbook of Clinical Specialties*, 5th edn. Oxford University Press, Oxford.

Glasier A. *et al.* (2000) *Handbook of Family Planning and Reproductive Healthcare*, 4th edn. Churchill Livingstone, London.

Hacker N.F. *et al.* (1998) *Essentials of Obstetrics and Gynaecology*. 3rd edn. W.B. Saunders Company, Philadelphia.

Paediatrics

Behrman R. *et al.* (1999) *Nelson's Textbook of Paediatrics*. W.B. Saunders, Philadelphia.

Lissauer T. (2001) *Illustrated Textbook of Paediatrics*. 2nd edn. Mosby, London.

In these questions candidates must select one answer only

Questions

1. A 50-year-old man complains of hardness of hearing and dyspnoea. He is noted to have a nasal septal perforation and a blood pressure of 140/90. His urinanalysis shows red cells, protein and casts. The chest x-ray reveals opacities. The most likely diagnosis is:

   A. tuberculosis
   B. amyloidosis
   C. Goodpasture's syndrome
   D. acute tubulointerstitial nephritis
   E. Wegener's granulomatosis

2. A football player presents with a drop foot after receiving a kick to his right leg. He can neither dorsiflex nor evert the foot. Sensation is lost over the front and outer half of the leg and dorsum of the foot. The most likely diagnosis is:

   A. superficial peroneal nerve injury
   B. common peroneal nerve injury
   C. tibial nerve injury
   D. lateral popliteal nerve
   E. sural nerve injury

3. A 50-year-old man with IDDM presents with a unilateral facial nerve palsy and severe earache. On auroscopic examination, he has granulation tissue deep in the external auditory meatus. The most likely diagnosis is:

   A. Bell's palsy
   B. sarcoidosis
   C. facial nerve schwannoma
   D. otitis externa complicated by local osteomyelitis (malignant otitis externa)
   E. suppurative otitis media

4. A 70-year-old woman presents with recent onset of urinary incontinence. The most appropriate initial investigation is:

A. MSU for dipstick
B. urodynamics
C. FBC
D. serum urea and electrolytes
E. MSU for culture and sensitivities

5. A 50-year-old woman with NIDDM presents with fever and a dusky red erythematous eruption over the left side of her face. The most likely organism would be:

A. *Staphylococcus aureus*
B. group B streptococcus
C. group A streptococcus
D. herpes zoster virus
E. herpes simplex virus

6. A 40-year-old woman presents with weight gain and depression. Her blood pressure is 150/90 and she has glycosuria. She complains also of secondary amenorrhoea and hirsutism. The most appropriate initial investigation would be:

A. 24-hour urine collection for urine-free cortisol assay
B. overnight dexamethasone suppression test
C. serum luteinising hormone and follicule stimulating hormone levels
D. serum testosterone
E. HbA1C

7. A 44-year-old woman complains of headaches and nosebleeds. Blood pressure is 160/100 in the right arm and 130/80 in the left arm. She complains of cold legs and has delayed radiofemoral pulses. The most likely diagnosis would be:

A. acromegaly
B. Marfan's syndrome
C. coarctation of the aorta
D. Kawasaki's disease
E. Takayusi's arteritis

8. A 55-year-old farmer complains of dry cough, exertional dyspnoea, joint pains and weight loss. He is noted to have finger clubbing. On x-ray there is bilateral diffuse reticulon-odular shadowing at the bases. The most likely diagnosis is:

A. bronchial carcinoma
B. bronchiectasis
C. cryptogenic fibrosing alveolitis
D. mesothelioma
E. extrinsic allergic alveolitis

9. A 45-year-old woman presents with pruritus and jaundice. She complains of dry eyes and mouth. The most discriminating investigation would be:

A. mitochondrial antibodies
B. anti-nuclear antibody
C. serum bilirubin and liver function tests
D. HBs antigen
E. smooth muscle antibody

10. An 80-year-old woman complains of sudden painless loss of vision in her right eye. She has facial pain on chewing. The most likely diagnosis is:

A. acute glaucoma
B. retinal detachment
C. cranial arteritis
D. basilar migraine
E. optic neuritis

11. A 13-year-old girl presents with a painful and swollen knee. There is no history of trauma. A tender lump is palpated over the tibial tuberosity. The most likely diagnosis would be:

A. osteomyelitis
B. chondromalacia patella
C. juvenile rheumatoid arthritis
D. osteosarcoma
E. Osgood–Schlatter disease

12. A 65-year-old man with NIDDM presents with a painless distended bladder. His urine dipstick shows no evidence of infection. The most useful investigation is:

    A. excretion urography
    B. retrograde ureterography
    C. serum urea and electrolytes
    D. cystourethroscopy
    E. pressure-flow studies

13. An 18-year-old known asthmatic presents with severe wheezing and a respiratory rate of 30 and a pulse of 120. She is using her accessory muscles and appears distressed. She is apyrexial. The most appropriate initial management would be:

    A. IM epinephrine (adrenaline)
    B. oxygen and nebulised salbutamol
    C. IV dexamethasone
    D. endotracheal intubation
    E. IV penicillin

14. A 25-year-old woman is brought to Casualty by ambulance having sustained gross maxillofacial deformities following a high speed RTA. She is now agitated and hypoxic despite high-concentration oxygen having been administered by face mask by the paramedics. The most appropriate immediate intervention is:

    A. endotracheal intubation
    B. nasopharyngeal airway
    C. oropharyngeal airway
    D. cricothyroidotomy
    E. laryngeal mask airway

15. A 14-year-old boy with cystic fibrosis presents with pneumonia. He also suffers from mild renal failure. The most appropriate antibiotic treatment is:

    A. tobramycin and carbenecillin
    B. ciprofloxacin
    C. tetracycline
    D. erythromycin
    E. cephalosporin

16. A 50-year-old woman who underwent a thyroidectomy a week ago now presents with confusion. She also complains of perioral tingling. The most discriminating investigation is:

A. serum glucose
B. LFTs
C. FBC and film
D. thyroid function tests
E. serum calcium

17. A 40-year-old man presents with progressive confusion and tremor. On examination, he has extensor plantar reflexes. The most useful investigation would be:

A. HIV serology
B. CT scan
C. drug levels
D. Mantoux test
E. VDRL

18. A 45-year-old man with a history of epilepsy presents with several weeks of fluctuating levels of consciousness. On examination his pupils are unequal. The most discriminating investigation is:

A. HIV serology
B. CT scan
C. electroencephalogram
D. drug levels
E. lumbar puncture

19. A 20-year-old heroin addict presents with weight loss, diarrhoea and confusion. On examination he has purple papules on his legs. The most useful investigation is:

A. echocardiogram
B. blood cultures
C. HIV serology
D. chest x-ray
E. drug levels

20. A 70-year-old man with alcohol dependence presents with sudden onset of productive purulent cough. The chest x-ray shows consolidation of the left upper lobe. The most likely pathogen is:

A. *Staphylococcus aureus*
B. *Streptococcus pneumoniae*
C. *Klebsiella pneumoniae*
D. *Mycoplasma pneumoniae*
E. *Pseudomonas aeruginosa*

21. A 60-year-old man presents with acute onset of confusion and restlessness; he walks with a broad-based gait. On examination there is nystagmus and lateral rectus palsies bilaterally. There is alcoholic foetor. The most likely diagnosis would be:

A. alcohol withdrawal
B. folic acid deficiency
C. subarachnoid haemorrhage
D. subdural haematoma
E. Wernicke–Korsakoff syndrome

22. A 40-year-old woman complains of disabling joint pains. On examination you note scaly plaques over her anterior shins and knees. She has tried diclofenac for the arthralgia and wonders if there is any connection with the rash. The most useful treatment for her joints now would be:

A. oral prednisolone
B. methotrexate
C. co-dydramol
D. topical 0.5% hydrocortisone
E. dithranol 0.1% cream

23. A 50-year-old man presents to Accident and Emergency complaining of 30 minutes of severe crushing mid-chest pain with no relief from GTN. He has a history of angina. Pulse is 105 and BP 115/60. 12-lead ECG shows normal sinus rhythm. The first drug to administer would be:

A. morphine
B. oxygen
C. gaviscon
D. streptokinase
E. atropine

24. A 40-year-old woman with a history of angina presents with severe chest pain for 30 minutes. Pulse is 45 and blood pressure 80/60. 12-lead ECG shows third-degree heart block. The first drug to administer would be:

    A. lidocaine (lignocaine)
    B. atropine
    C. epinephrine (adrenaline)
    D. procainamide
    E. amiodarone

25. A 40-year-old patient is brought to Casualty by ambulance in pulseless electrical activity (PEA). You are told he was given epinephrine (adrenaline). The next step would be to:

    A. evaluate for reversible causes
    B. defibrillate with 200 J
    C. administer verapamil
    D. administer amiodarone
    E. administer morphine

26. A 70-year-old woman presents with progressive dysphagia and food regurgitation. On examination she has halitosis and a small lump on the left side of her neck. The most likely diagnosis is:

    A. achalasia
    B. branchial cyst
    C. diffuse oesophageal spasm
    D. pharyngeal pouch
    E. myasthenia gravis

27. A 20-year-old slightly withdrawn man states he experiences auditory hallucinations. He is noted to have poverty of speech and a flat affect. The most likely diagnosis would be:

    A. schizophrenia
    B. manic-depressive disorder
    C. delirium
    D. dementia
    E. opioid abuse

28. A 50-year-old man complains of loss of libido. He takes Humulin and Actrapid insulin. He is noted to have an enlarged liver. The most discriminating investigation is:

    A. serum copper and caeruloplasmin
    B. serum gamma-glutamyl transferase
    C. HbsAg
    D. serum iron and total iron binding capacity
    E. mitochondrial antibodies

29. A 40-year-old woman presents with fatigue, dyspnoea and paraesthesiae. On examination she has a red tongue. Blood film shows hypersegmented neutrophils, a Hb of 9 and an MCV of 120 fl. The most likely diagnosis is:

    A. vitamin B_{12} deficiency
    B. iron deficiency
    C. coeliac disease
    D. sideroblastic anaemia
    E. hypothyroidism

30. An 18-year-old female, who recently started the combined oral contraceptive pill on holiday in Kenya, complains of colicky abdominal pain, vomiting and fever. Urine is positive for red blood cells and protein. She develops progressive weakness in her extremities. The most likely diagnosis is:

    A. acute pyelonephritis
    B. acute intermittent porphyria
    C. ureteric calculus
    D. malaria
    E. systemic lupus erythematosus

31. An 87-year-old man is noted to have an altered level of consciousness. The serum glucose is 37 mmol/L with a serum sodium of 163 mmol/L. He has no prior history of diabetes. He has been on intravenous fluids for a week with IV cefuroxime and metronidazole for a chest infection. The most appropriate treatment would be:

    A. insulin sliding scale, heparin and 0.45% normal saline
    B. insulin sliding scale, heparin and 0.9% saline
    C. insulin sliding scale, 0.9% normal saline
    D. insulin sliding scale, 0.45% normal saline
    E. insulin sliding scale, dextrose saline

32. A 40-year-old actor with IDDM is started on propranolol for stage fright. He collapses on stage. He has not changed his insulin regime. Serum glucose is 1.5 mmol/L. The most beneficial advice you would offer him after treatment would be:

   A. discontinue propranolol
   B. carry a chocolate bar
   C. decrease his Humulin insulin
   D. decrease his Actrapid insulin
   E. carry glucagon

33. A 40-year-old woman complains of intolerance to cold weather and cold running water. On examination you note she has a beaked nose, radial furrowing of the lips and facial telangiectasiae. On examination of her hands you notice sausage-like digits and tapered fingers. The most discriminating investigation to establish her diagnosis is:

   A. anticentromere antinuclear antibody
   B. rheumatoid factor
   C. FBC
   D. chest x-ray
   E. barium swallow

34. A 60-year-old woman presents with a slow-growing, painless but itchy flat red scaly plaque on her lateral lower calf. The most useful investigation would be:

   A. skin scrapings
   B. skin biopsy
   C. serum glucose
   D. none – spot diagnosis
   E. sentinel node biopsy

35. Stevens–Johnson syndrome is associated with all of the following drugs EXCEPT:

   A. penicillin
   B. sulphonamides
   C. oral contraceptives
   D. thiazide diuretics
   E. salicylates

36. A 65-year-old farmer presents with a grey thickened patch of skin on the rim of his left ear. The 1-cm lesion is painless, raised, firm, and has not changed in size over many years. The most likely diagnosis is:

   A. basal cell carcinoma
   B. keratoacanthoma
   C. solar keratosis
   D. seborrhoeic keratosis
   E. squamous cell carcinoma

37. A 55-year-old woman complains of sudden severe central abdominal pain radiating to her back and vomiting. She prefers to sit forwards on her stretcher. Temperature is 39°C, BP 100/60 and pulse 112. On examination she has a markedly tender epigastrium and a bruise over the left flank. She has a history of gallstones. She denies smoking or alcohol. She takes HRT. The most discriminating investigation would be:

   A. plain abdominal x-ray
   B. serum bilirubin and liver function tests
   C. serum amylase
   D. FBC
   E. abdominal ultrasound

38. A 60-year-old man presents with increasing abdominal girth. On examination you elicit shifting dullness. You decide to obtain an ascitic fluid tap. The following should be routinely requested on the fluid EXCEPT:

   A. cell count
   B. Gram stain and culture for bacteria and AFB
   C. albumin and protein
   D. cytology
   E. glucose

39. A 60-year-old man with essential hypertension presents with right painful eye. On examination he is noted to have right partial ptosis and right fixed dilated pupil. The eye is looking downwards and outwards. The most likely diagnosis is:

   A. trochlear nerve palsy
   B. abducens nerve palsy
   C. incomplete oculomotor nerve palsy
   D. posterior communicating artery aneurysm
   E. optic neuritis

40. A 40-year-old man with IDDM complains of seeing flashing lights and floaters in his eyes. On examination he is noted to have a unilateral irregular field defect. The most likely diagnosis is:

A. migraine with focal aura
B. vitreous haemorrhage
C. retinal detachment
D. acute angle closure glaucoma
E. central retinal artery occlusion

41. A 17-year-old boy presents with pain on swallowing. On examination he has trismus, palatal petechiae and enlarged tonsils. His sclerae are jaundiced. The most likely causative organism is:

A. *Streptococcus pneumoniae*
B. hepatitis B virus
C. Epstein–Barr virus
D. herpes simplex virus
E. *Clostridium tetani*

42. A 20-year-old woman presents with recurrent epistaxis. She admits to having heavy periods. BP is 90/60 and pulse 100. There are bruises of different ages over her extremities but no splenomegaly. Test results are as follows:

white cell count	8×10^9/L
Hb	11.5 g/dL
platelets	20×10^9/L
bleeding time	prolonged
antinuclear antibody	negative

The most likely diagnosis is:

A. non-accidental injury
B. systemic lupus erythematosus
C. chronic idiopathic thrombocytopenia
D. thrombotic thrombocytopenic purpura
E. sickle-cell disease

43. A 45-year-old woman presents with severe itching, recent pale stools and dark urine. On examination there is darkened skin pigmentation, xanthelasma and hepatomegaly. Test results are as follows:

serum bilirubin	15 μmol/L
serum alkaline phosphatase	400 IU/L (30–300 IU/L)
AST	40 IU/L (5–35 IU/L)

Diagnosis would best be confirmed by:

A. serum antimitochondrial antibody
B. hepatitis virology
C. liver biopsy
D. Kveim test
E. abdominal ultrasound

44. A 60-year-old man presents with increasing abdominal girth. On examination you elicit shifting dullness. The ascitic fluid tap reveals straw-coloured fluid containing 50 g/L of protein and elevated LDH. It contains 1000 WBCs/mm^3 (no lymphocytes) and many red cells are present. Serum total protein is 40 g/L. The most likely diagnosis is:

A. cirrhosis
B. tuberculosis
C. malignancy
D. pancreatitis
E. hepatic vein obstruction

45. A 55-year-old man complains of rectal bleeding. He is noted to have freckles on his lips. His father also has freckles on the lips and underwent bowel surgery but he is not sure why. The most likely diagnosis is:

A. Crohn's disease
B. ulcerative colitis
C. Peutz–Jegher syndrome
D. hereditary haemorrhagic telangiectasia
E. familial adenomatous polyposis

46. A 40-year-old longstay patient in a psychiatric hospital presents with fever, abdominal pain, dry cough and worsening confusion. Blood tests reveal neutrophilia, lymphopenia and hyponatraemia. Chest x-ray shows right-sided lobar consolidation. The most likely diagnosis is:

    A. tuberculosis
    B. streptococcus pneumonia
    C. legionella pneumonia
    D. klebsiella pneumonia
    E. staphylococcus pneumonia

47. A 50-year-old man with schizophrenia presents with drooling saliva and involuntary chewing movements. He walks with a shuffling gait. The most likely diagnosis is:

    A. Parkinson's disease
    B. extrapyramidal side-effect of medication
    C. autonomic side-effect of medication
    D. anticholinergic side-effect of medication
    E. lithium toxicity

48. A 40-year-old man presents with numbness and tingling sensation in his feet. He is noted to have distal sensory loss and absent ankle jerk reflexes. The knee-jerk reflexes are exaggerated. He drinks heavily and smokes cigars. Blood pressure 160/90 with a pulse of 90. Full blood count reveals a macrocytic megaloblastic anaemia. The most likely diagnosis is:

    A. syringomyelia
    B. tabes dorsalis
    C. Wernicke–Korsakoff syndrome
    D. vitamin B_6 deficiency
    E. subacute combined degeneration of the cord

49. The following statements regarding testicular tumours are correct EXCEPT:

    A. Seminomas usually present in men in their forties.
    B. Teratomas are radiosensitive.
    C. Cryptorchism is a risk factor.
    D. The contralateral testicle should be biopsied, if there is a history of infertility.
    E. After orchidectomy the disease is staged by chest and abdominal CT scan.

50. A 40-year-old woman presents with a right-sided pleural effusion and ascites. Abdominal ultrasound reveals a left ovarian mass. The most likely diagnosis is:

    A. pseudomyxoma peritonei
    B. Meig's syndrome
    C. Budd–Chiari syndrome
    D. nephrotic syndrome
    E. tuberculosis

51. A 30-year-old man presents with a tender swollen testicle. He states that he was bumped in the groin while playing sports. On examination the borders of the testicle are irregular, and the testicle is heavy and woody. There is no associated lymphadenopathy. He is also noted to have gynaecomastia. There are no external signs of trauma. In this age group, the most likely diagnosis is:

    A. testicular torsion
    B. epididymo-orchitis
    C. seminoma
    D. teratoma
    E. testicular haematoma

52. A 45-year-old male psychiatric patient with long-term bipolar disorder presents with vomiting, muscle twitching and tremor. He was started on bendrofluazide recently and self-prescribes ibuprofen for headaches. BP 90/50. His gait is ataxic. He then starts fitting. The drug most likely to be responsible is:

    A. lithium
    B. phenothiazine
    C. benzodiazepine
    D. ecstasy (MDMA)
    E. ibuprofen

53. A 60-year-old man presents acutely with vertigo and vomiting. On neurological examination there is right facial numbness, an ipsilateral ataxia of arm and leg is present and a contralateral loss of pain and temperature sense. The most likely diagnosis is:

    A. posterior cerebral artery infarction
    B. middle cerebral artery infarction
    C. anterior cerebral artery infarction
    D. posterior inferior cerebellar artery infarction
    E. vertebrobasilar ischaemia

54. A 60-year-old man presents with persistent fever, profuse watery diarrhoea and crampy abdominal pain for the past week. He has just completed treatment for osteomyelitis. Proctosigmoidoscopy reveals erythematous ulcerations and yellowish-white plaques. The most likely diagnosis is:

    A. ulcerative colitis
    B. Crohn's disease
    C. pseudomembranous colitis
    D. viral gastroenteritis
    E. *Clostridium perfringens* enterocolitis

55. You are on ward rounds and notice that a young patient is coughing briskly. He has just been commenced on benzylpenicillin for acute tonsillitis complicated by trismus. He states he does not know if he is allergic to any drugs. He becomes short of breath. Pulse is 110 beats/minute and he now cannot complete sentences. The most appropriate management for this patient would be:

    A. administer epinephrine (adrenaline) of a 1 : 10 000 solution intravenously
    B. administer epinephrine (adrenaline) intramuscularly for suspected new-onset asthma
    C. administer oxygen and give nebulised salbutamol
    D. administer oxygen and epinephrine (adrenaline) of a 1 : 1000 solution intramuscularly for suspected anaphylaxis
    E. administer oxygen and give IV hydrocortisone for anaphylactic shock

56. A 45-year-old obese man is noted to have glycosuria. He has no symptoms. Diabetes is confirmed on oral glucose tolerance test. The most appropriate management for this patient is:

   A. commence biguanide
   B. commence sulphonylurea
   C. advise on diet and exercise
   D. commence on Humulin and Actrapid insulin
   E. admit to hospital

57. A 45-year-old well-controlled insulin-dependent diabetic is prescribed captopril for hypertension. He has a history of intermittent claudication and suffers rest pain. There is 3+ proteinuria. Urea and creatinine are elevated. On examination there is an abdominal bruit. The most likely diagnosis is:

   A. diabetic nephropathy
   B. focal segmental glomerulosclerosis
   C. renal artery stenosis
   D. membranous glomerulonephritis
   E. renal cholesterol embolism

58. A 20-year-old man presents with buttock pain radiating down both legs and heel pain. On examination he has marked kyphosis and limitation of chest expansion. ESR and CRP were raised. The most likely diagnosis is:

   A. lumbar disc prolapse
   B. sacro-iliitis
   C. spondylolisthesis
   D. spinal stenosis
   E. ankylosing spondylitis

59. A 55-year-old man has been treated with three consecutive shocks of 200 J, 200 J and 360 J for ventricular fibrillation. The morphology of his rhythm does not change. The most appropriate next step in management is:

   A. administer 4th shock at 360 J immediately
   B. recheck pulse and administer 4th shock at 360 J
   C. recheck pulse and administer amiodarone 300 mg IV if the systolic BP is < 90
   D. recheck pulse and blood pressure, commence CPR and administer lidocaine (lignocaine) 50 mg if the systolic BP is < 90
   E. recheck pulse and blood pressure, commence CPR and administer amiodarone 300 mg IV if the systolic BP is > 90

60. The definitive investigation to diagnose a pulmonary embolism is:

A. arterial blood gases
B. ventilation-perfusion isotope scintigraphy
C. pulmonary angiogram
D. 12-lead electrocardiogram
E. PA and lateral chest x-ray

61. Which one of the following drugs is absolutely contraindicated in patients with asthma?

A. adenosine
B. atenolol
C. epinephrine (adrenaline)
D. verapamil
E. bendrofluazide

62. A 70-year-old man complains of flashing lights and floaters in his left eye for the past month and now complains of painless loss of vision in his left eye. The most likely diagnosis is:

A. central retinal artery occlusion
B. central retinal vein occlusion
C. optic neuritis
D. retinal detachment
E. macular degeneration

63. A 30-year-old man with HIV presents with sudden bilateral painless loss of vision. The most likely cause is:

A. Kaposi's sarcoma
B. candidiasis
C. *Chlamydia trachomatis*
D. CMV retinitis
E. gonococcal infection

64. A 50-year-old man presents to Casualty with repeated fits. Plasma sodium is 112 mmol/L and urine osmolality is 550 mmol/kg. He is well hydrated. On chest-x-ray there is a cannon-ball lesion. He smokes 20 cigarettes a day and drinks spirits daily. The most likely diagnosis is:

A. SIADH
B. Addison's disease
C. liver cirrhosis
D. renal failure
E. diabetes insipidus

65. A 60-year-old man has squamous cell carcinoma of the bronchus. The most useful investigation to assess curative surgical resection is:

A. radionucleotide scanning for the detection of metastatic disease
B. fibreoptic bronchoscopy and cytology
C. CT scan of the mediastinum
D. measurement of FEV_1
E. transthoracic fine-needle aspiration biopsy of mediastinal lymph node

66. A 60-year-old man presents with chest pain and sudden onset of atrial fibrillation with a heart rate of 160/min. The most appropriate management would be:

A. oxygen, heparin and synchronised DC shock
B. oxygen, heparin, IV amiodarone
C. oxygen, heparin, warfarin
D. oxygen, beta-blockers
E. oxygen, digoxin IV

67. A 65-year-old man presents with an acute myocardial infarction with a new left bundle branch block. He had a haemorrhagic stroke a year ago. He is given 100% oxygen, diamorphine, metoclopramide, GTN and aspirin. The next most appropriate management is:

A. IV glycoprotein IIb/IIIa inhibitor
B. thrombolytic therapy with streptokinase
C. coronary artery bypass surgery
D. percutaneous transluminal coronary angioplasty
E. continuous infusion of heparin

68. Which one of the following drugs may induce a psychosis similar to paranoid schizophrenia?

A. heroin
B. ecstasy (MDMA)
C. amphetamine
D. cocaine
E. barbiturates

69. A 50-year-old man presents with dyspnoea on exertion. On examination he is noted to have distended neck veins, hepatomegaly and ascites. He is also noted to have a paradoxical pulse and a rising JVP on inspiration. Chest x-ray reveals a small heart and calcification. The most likely diagnosis is:

A. viral pericarditis
B. tuberculous constrictive pericarditis
C. cardiac tamponade
D. malignant pericarditis
E. Dressler's syndrome

70. A 20-year-old woman presents with a BP of 170/100. On examination she has impalpable peripheral pulses, although systolic murmurs are auscultated above and below her clavicle. She also complains of diminishing vision and syncopal episodes. ESR is 50 mm/h. The most likely diagnosis is:

A. thrombangiitis obliterans
B. coarctation of the aorta
C. Kawasaki's disease
D. Takayasu's syndrome
E. Raynaud's disease

71. A 35-year-old IV drug abuser presents with right upper quadrant abdominal pain. On examination he has peripheral oedema, ascites and a pulsatile liver. On chest auscultation he has a pansystolic murmur along the left sternal border. The most likely diagnosis is:

A. tricuspid regurgitation
B. pulmonary regurgitation
C. pulmonary stenosis
D. mitral regurgitation
E. tricuspid stenosis

72. A 50-year-old woman presents with fever, headache, left eye pain and blurry vision. She states that she has just recovered from a cold. On examination she has a swollen left eyelid, mild proptosis and diminished visual acuity. She is unable to move her eye. The most likely diagnosis is:

A. orbital cellulitis
B. giant-cell arteritis
C. sinusitis
D. choroiditis
E. cavernous sinus thrombosis

73. A 60-year-old woman presents with progressive forgetfulness and mood changes. She has a shuffling gait. CT scan of the head shows cortical atrophy and enlarged ventricles. Histology shows senile plaques and neurofibrillary tangles. The most likely diagnosis is:

A. Wernicke–Korsakoff syndrome
B. Parkinson's disease
C. Alzheimer's disease
D. variant Creutzfeldt–Jakob disease
E. multi-infarct dementia

74. A 20-year-old college student presents with headache and dry cough. The chest x-ray shows left lower lobe consolidation. White cell count is normal. Cold agglutinins are detected. The most likely pathogen is:

A. *Streptococcus pneumoniae*
B. *Klebsiella* sp.
C. Mycoplasma
D. *Haemophilus influenzae*
E. *Legionella pneumophila*

75. A 25-year-old man presents with weakness and numbness in his lower legs. He has just recovered from a recent chest infection. On examination deep tendon reflexes are absent and sensation is also lost. CSF from a lumbar puncture shows a normal cell count and glucose but raised protein level. The most likely diagnosis is:

A. mumps
B. sarcoidosis
C. AIDS
D. Guillain–Barré syndrome
E. Refsum's disease

76. A 40-year-old man presents with dysphagia and epigastric pain relieved by food and antacids. On examination he has a palpable epigastric mass, a palpable supraclavicular lymph node and acanthosis nigricans. The most likely diagnosis is:

   A. oesophageal squamous cell carcinoma
   B. duodenal ulcer
   C. peptic stricture of oesophagogastric junction
   D. gastric adenocarcinoma
   E. pancreatic carcinoma

77. A 17-year-old girl presents with meningism and conjunctival petechiae. The CSF is turbid with an abundance of poly-morphs and protein. Gram-negative cocci are isolated. The most likely organism is:

   A. *Neisseria meningitidis*
   B. *Neisseria gonorrhoea*
   C. group B streptococcus
   D. *Haemophilus influenzae*
   E. *Streptococcus pneumoniae*

78. A 22-year-old male presents with fever, sweating particularly at night, pruritus and weight loss. On examination he has palpable painless cervical lymph nodes and no skin manifes-tations. The most appropriate investigation would be:

   A. FBC
   B. lymph node biopsy
   C. chest x-ray
   D. CT scan of neck and mediastinum
   E. Mantoux test

79. The most likely diagnosis is:

   A. tuberculosis
   B. non-Hodgkin's lymphoma
   C. Hodgkin's lymphoma
   D. acute lymphoblastic leukaemia
   E. chronic lymphocytic leukaemia

80. A 40-year-old woman complains of intolerance to cold weather and cold running water. On examination you note she has a beaked nose, radial furrowing of the lips and facial telangiectasiae. On examination of her hands you notice sausage-like digits and tapered fingers. The most likely diagnosis is:

A. SLE
B. Sjögren's syndrome
C. systemic sclerosis
D. rheumatoid arthritis
E. dermatomyositis

81. A 50-year-old renal transplant recipient on immunosuppressive therapy with cyclosporin, azathioprine and prednisolone is most at risk of developing:

A. squamous cell carcinoma of the skin
B. basal cell carcinoma of the skin
C. lymphoma
D. liver failure
E. leukaemia

82. You are called to see a 65-year-old woman for poor urine output. She is on IV flucloxacillin, benzylpenicillin and metronidazole for pelvic cellulitis. A Foley bladder catheter is inserted and the hourly urine output is confirmed as 10 ml/hour. Temperature is 38°C, blood pressure 160/90 and pulse rate 110. ECG shows peaked T waves and wide QRS complexes. Blood results include:

plasma sodium	139 mmol/L
plasma potassium	6.9 mmol/L
plasma urea	12 mmol/L
plasma creatinine	300 μmol/L

The most appropriate management for this patient is:

A. administer a bolus of 1 litre of Hartmann's solution
B. administer 10% calcium gluconate slowly into a central vein and administer 50 ml of 50% dextrose with 10 units of soluble human insulin over 30 minutes
C. administer $NaHCO_3$ slowly IV into a central vein
D. administer 120 mg furosemide (frusemide) as a bolus dose IV
E. take blood cultures

83. A 25-year-old man presents to Casualty with repeated fits. He smells of alcohol and has jaw trismus. The most appropriate management is:

   A. give 100 mg of IV thiamine
   B. give 50 ml of 50% glucose IV
   C. give 10 mg IV diazepam over 2 minutes
   D. insert a Guedel oropharyngeal airway and prepare for endotracheal intubation
   E. insert a nasopharyngeal airway and administer oxygen

84. A 40-year-old man presents to Casualty within 1 hour of a paracetamol overdose. He smells of alcohol. His family confirms that he drinks heavily but is not on any medication. 16 tablets are missing from his paracetamol packs. The most appropriate management would be:

   A. take emergency blood levels for paracetamol level
   B. give oral DL-methionine immediately followed by activated charcoal
   C. administer activated charcoal first
   D. give IV N-acetylcysteine in 5% dextrose over 15 minutes
   E. no treatment is required

85. A 55-year-old man presents with an acutely painful swollen right knee. He was recently prescribed bendrofluazide for mild hypertension. The most useful investigation would be:

   A. FBC and ESR
   B. viral antibodies including parvovirus
   C. anti-nuclear antibody and rheumatoid factor
   D. aspirate of joint effusion for gram stain and culture
   E. aspirate of joint effusion for polarised light microscopy

86. A 17-year-old man with known sickle-cell disease presents with severe lower back pain. He has a history of seizures. Initial management should be:

   A. give oxygen at 4 L/min via a face mask
   B. start IV fluids
   C. give pethidine 150 mg IM every 2 hours until the pain settles
   D. give morphine 1–2 mg IV every 2–3 minutes until the pain settles
   E. lumbar spine and pelvic x-ray

87. A 55-year-old intoxicated man is brought to Casualty by the police. He is confused and aggressive. There are no external signs of head trauma. BP is 140/90, heart rate 110 and he is pale. He has palmar erythema, tremors and smells of alcohol. The most useful investigation for this man is:

A. blood alcohol level
B. head CT scan
C. gamma glutamyl transferase
D. blood glucose
E. clotting screen

88. A 25-year-old man presents to Casualty with sudden onset of severe lower back pain that radiates down his right leg. On examination he is noted to have scoliosis of the spine, limited spinal flexion, restricted straight-leg raise, limited hip movements and sensory loss over the dorsum of the right foot. The most likely diagnosis is:

A. spondylolisthesis
B. ankylosing spondylitis
C. acute cord compression
D. spondylosis
E. lumbar disc prolapse

89. A 35-year-old man presents with progressive weakness in his limbs over the past few days. He had a chest infection 2 weeks prior. On examination he has proximal muscle wasting, hypotonia and absent deep tendon reflexes. Lumbar puncture results are:

cells	4/cc lymphocytes
chloride	110 mmol/L
glucose	3.5 mmol/L
protein	3 g/L

The most likely diagnosis is:

A. poliomyelitis
B. botulism
C. Guillain–Barré syndrome
D. AIDS
E. subacute combined degeneration of the cord

90. The most useful step in guiding management would be:

    A. pulse oximetry
    B. chest x-ray
    C. nerve conduction studies
    D. serial vital capacity
    E. serial peak flow measurement

91. A 50-year-old obese man presents complaining of recurrent abdominal pain radiating to the back and made worse by eating and bending over. Antacids relieve the pain. He smokes 20 cigarettes a day and drinks spirits daily. The most useful investigation would be:

    A. oesophagogastroduodenoscopy
    B. double contrast barium meal
    C. *Helicobacter pylori* breath test
    D. abdominal x-ray
    E. abdominal CT scan

92. The most likely diagnosis is:

    A. duodenal ulcer
    B. gastro-oesophageal reflux disease
    C. acute pancreatitis
    D. achalasia
    E. Barrett's ulcer of the oesophagus

93. A 30-year-old man presents with crampy abdominal pain, diarrhoea and weight loss. On examination: temperature 39°C; no lymphadenopathy. Barium meal reveals a stricture in the terminal ileum. The most likely diagnosis is:

    A. tuberculosis
    B. Crohn's disease
    C. ulcerative colitis
    D. lymphoma
    E. coeliac disease

94. A 30-year-old man presents with a unilateral facial nerve palsy that involves his forehead. Possible causes include the following EXCEPT:

A. Bell's palsy
B. Ramsay–Hunt syndrome
C. acoustic neuroma
D. cerebrovascular accident
E. parotid tumour

95. On general examination the man has coarse oily skin and a prominent supraorbital ridge. He has widely spaced teeth and a moist handshake. The man's general appearance is suspicious of:

A. acromegaly
B. haemochromatosis
C. Klinefelter's syndrome
D. gigantism
E. Hurler's syndrome

96. A 50-year-old man presents with a lump in the posterior triangle of the neck. It has been present for 8 months and is associated with a cheesy serous discharge. The most likely diagnosis is:

A. squamous cell carcinoma
B. tuberculous adenitis
C. deep lobe of parotid tumour
D. infected branchial cyst
E. infected lymph node

97. Prophylaxis against opportunistic infections is advised when the CD4 count falls below:

A. 500 cells/mm^3
B. 300 cells/mm^3
C. 250 cells/mm^3
D. 200 cells/mm^3
E. 100 cells/mm^3

98. All the following are opportunistic infections in HIV disease EXCEPT:

A. *Mycobacterium avium*
B. *Toxoplasma gondii*
C. *Pneumocystis carinii*
D. cytomegalovirus
E. *Helicobacter pylori*

99. Recognised side-effects of heparin include the following EXCEPT:

A. thrombosis
B. thrombocytopenia
C. alopecia
D. osteoporosis
E. hypokalaemia

100. The following statements regarding anorexia nervosa are true EXCEPT:

A. A BMI < 13 warrants hospital admission.
B. Anorexia is defined as a BMI < 17.5 associated with food avoidance.
C. Physical features include bradycardia and hypotension.
D. Investigations are important in confirming the diagnosis.
E. Anorexia may be associated with reduced bone mass.

101. The most useful initial screening test for SLE is:

A. anti-dsDNA antibody
B. anti-nuclear antibody
C. anti-cardiolipin antibody
D. C3 and C4 levels
E. anti-extractable nuclear antigen (ENA) antibody

102. Rheumatoid arthritis may be associated with all of the following EXCEPT:

A. ulnar drift deformity
B. carpal tunnel syndrome
C. Dupuytren's contracture
D. painful flexor tenosynovitis
E. trigger finger

103. Carpal tunnel syndrome is associated with all of the following EXCEPT:

A. degenerative arthritis
B. pregnancy
C. acromegaly
D. Colles' fracture
E. diabetes

104. A 30-year-old female involved in a road traffic accident is brought by ambulance to Casualty. She is noted to have bruising over the mastoid process and periorbital haematoma. On otoscopic examination she has bleeding behind the tympanic membrane. The most likely diagnosis is:

A. extradural haematoma
B. subdural haematoma
C. basal skull fracture
D. depressed occipital skull fracture
E. intracerebral haemorrhage

105. A 54-year-old man with IDDM presents with fever, and a painful and swollen right lower leg. On examination, the pulses are absent distally, the foot cold and subcutaneous crepitus is present. The most useful investigation is:

A. x-ray of the leg
B. Doppler ultrasound
C. arteriogram
D. blood cultures
E. venogram

106. The most likely diagnosis is:

A. osteomyelitis
B. gas gangrene
C. chronic ischaemia of the leg
D. deep venous thrombosis
E. acute ischaemia of the leg

107. A 45-year-old woman presents with pruritus, pale stools and dark urine. On examination she has finger clubbing and hepatosplenomegaly. Blood tests reveal a normal bilirubin, elevated alkaline phosphatase and low T4. The most certain way to confirm the diagnosis is by:

    A. anti-mitochondrial antibody
    B. liver biopsy
    C. ERCP
    D. CT scan of the abdomen
    E. hepatitis A, B and C serology

108. A 70-year-old man, who lives alone and is self-caring, presents with weakness in his lower legs and muscle pain. On examination he has loose teeth and is noted to have ecchymoses of the lower limbs. He suffers from rheumatoid arthritis, which greatly limits his mobility. The most likely diagnosis is:

    A. folate deficiency
    B. scurvy
    C. iron deficiency
    D. thiamine deficiency
    E. vitamin B_{12} deficiency

109. A 20-year-old man presents with persistent eye irritation. He explains that he is sensitive to light, has noted worsening vision and complains of aching eyes. He also complains of morning stiffness in his back. The most likely diagnosis is:

    A. keratitis
    B. uveitis
    C. viral conjunctivitis
    D. episcleritis
    E. choroiditis

110. The most useful investigation for this man would be:

    A. lumbar and pelvic spine x-ray
    B. Kveim test
    C. HIV test
    D. Mantoux test
    E. rheumatoid factor

111. Which one of the following drugs CANNOT be administered via the tracheal route?

A. epinephrine (adrenaline)
B. atropine
C. amiodarone
D. lidocaine (lignocaine)
E. naloxone

112. The following statements regarding Good Medical Practice are correct EXCEPT:

A. You must provide the necessary care to alleviate pain and distress whether or not curative treatment is possible.
B. You may end a professional relationship with a patient if he or she makes a complaint about you or your team.
C. In an emergency, wherever it may arise, you must offer anyone at risk the assistance you could reasonably be expected to provide.
D. You must respond constructively to the outcome of appraisals of your performance.
E. You must take part in adverse event recognition and reporting to help reduce risk to patients.

113. Diagnostic features of post-traumatic stress disorder include all of the following EXCEPT:

A. autonomic arousal
B. recurrent, obtrusive thoughts
C. symptoms of anxiety
D. memory impairment
E. loss of orientation

114. Diagnostic features of panic disorder include all of the following EXCEPT:

A. dizziness
B. feelings of unreality
C. fear of insanity
D. fear of leaving home
E. choking sensations

115. Diagnostic features of mania include all of the following EXCEPT:

   A. labile mood
   B. rapid speech
   C. loss of inhibitions
   D. overeating
   E. grandiosity

116. A 35-year-old African woman is found to have a Hb of 6 g/dL. She is a vegetarian and has a history of uterine fibroids. Blood film reveals microcytic, hypochromic red blood cells and a few target cells. The most likely diagnosis is:

   A. thalassaemia trait
   B. iron-deficiency anaemia
   C. sickle-cell disease
   D. anaemia of chronic disease
   E. sideroblastic anaemia

117. A 25-year-old woman presents with a single, non-tender enlarged cervical lymph node. She also complains of fever and night sweats. Lymph node biopsy reveals infiltration with histiocytes and lymphocytes and the presence of cells with bilobed mirror-image nuclei. The most likely diagnosis is:

   A. non-Hodgkin's lymphoma
   B. Hodgkin's lymphoma
   C. sarcoidosis
   D. acute lymphoblastic leukaemia
   E. tuberculosis

118. A 45-year-old woman with diabetes presents with shiny waxy erythematous plaques on her shins with yellowish skin and telangiectasia. The most likely diagnosis is:

   A. pretibial myxoedema
   B. pyoderma gangrenosum
   C. psoriasis
   D. erythema nodosum
   E. necrobiosis lipoidica

119. A 40-year-old man is brought to Casualty in a comatose state. Useful initial investigations include all of the following EXCEPT:

A. serum glucose
B. serum calcium
C. arterial blood gases
D. FBC
E. blood alcohol level

120. On examination he is noted to have constricted pupils and depressed respirations. The most appropriate management would be:

A. head CT scan
B. naloxone 0.4–1.2 mg IV stat
C. flumazenil 200 µg IV over 15 seconds
D. doxapram IV
E. dantrolene 1 mg/kg IV

121. A 55-year-old man complains of generalised weakness for the past month. He also complains of excessive thirst and frequent micturition. Blood results:

urine glucose	negative
urine nitrate	negative
serum creatinine	140 µmol/L
serum urea	10 mmol/L
serum calcium	3.5 mmol/L
serum phosphate	1 mmol/L
serum alkaline phosphatase	200 IU/L (30–300 IU/L)
serum albumin	45 g/L

These findings are consistent with all of the following diseases EXCEPT:

A. primary hyperparathyroidism
B. sarcoidosis
C. multiple myeloma
D. thyrotoxicosis
E. bone metastases

122. The following are useful investigations to establish the diagnosis EXCEPT:

A. FBC
B. chest x-ray
C. ESR
D. parathyroid hormone
E. magnesium

123. Chest x-ray reveals bilateral hilar lymphadenopathy. The most likely diagnosis is:

A. multiple myeloma
B. sarcoidosis
C. primary hyperparathyroidism
D. bone metastases
E. thyrotoxicosis

124. A 60-year-old man presents to Casualty with painless profuse haematuria for the past 2 days. On examination BP 90/50 and pulse 105/min. Blood results:

white cell count	5×10^9/L
Hb	6 g/dL
platelets	150×10^9/L
serum creatinine	300 µmol/L
serum urea	20 mmol/L

Following resuscitation, the patient is no longer bleeding. The most useful investigation would be:

A. cystoscopy
B. intravenous pyelogram
C. ultrasound of the kidneys, bladder and prostate
D. pelvic CT scan
E. retrograde urography

125. A 25-year-old woman presents to the outpatient clinic with a neck swelling. On examination the swelling moves upward with protrusion of the tongue. The most likely diagnosis is:

A. thyroid goitre
B. cystic hygroma
C. thyroglossal cyst
D. branchial cyst
E. thyroid malignancy

126. A 20-year-old man arrives in Casualty with marked dys-
     pnoea; he suffers from asthma. On examination respiratory
     rate 24/min and pulse 105/min. Peak flow is 60% of pre-
     dicted. The most appropriate management would be:

     A. treat in casualty with nebulised salbutamol 5 mg and repeat peak
        flow in 30 minutes
     B. arrange immediate hospital admission and treat with IV hydro-
        cortisone 200 mg
     C. arrange immediate hospital admission, administer oxygen 40–60%,
        nebulised salbutamol and oral prednisolone 30–60 mg
     D. arrange immediate hospital admission, administer oxygen-driven
        nebuliser and give slow IV aminophylline 250 mg
     E. treat in Casualty with oral prednisolone 30–60 mg and repeat peak
        flow in 30 minutes

127. A 55-year-old smoker with a history of chronic productive
     cough presents to Casualty breathless and drowsy. On exam-
     ination he is centrally cyanosed with a raised JVP and a pal-
     pable liver. There is a blowing pansystolic murmur at the
     lower left sternal border. No abnormality is heard in the
     lungs. The most likely diagnosis is:

     A. infective endocarditis
     B. cor pulmonale
     C. rheumatic heart disease
     D. exacerbation of chronic bronchitis
     E. emphysema

128. The most useful diagnostic investigation is:

     A. arterial blood gas
     B. 12-lead electrocardiogram
     C. lung function tests
     D. chest x-ray
     E. sputum examination

129. The most appropriate treatment is:

     A. continuous oxygen therapy
     B. furosemide (frusemide)
     C. salbutamol inhaler
     D. oral prednisolone 30 mg od
     E. amoxicillin 500 mg o tds

130. A 20-year-old man is found unconscious after a night of binge drinking. There is no evidence of physical trauma. On examination he has alcohol on his breath and a bitten tongue. Blood pressure 110/80 and pulse 80/min. The pupils are small, equal and responsive to light. On removal of his clothes, his trousers are noted to be soiled with urine. The most likely suspicion is:

   A. hypoglycaemic coma
   B. alcoholic overdose
   C. postictal phase of an epileptic seizure
   D. subarachnoid haemorrhage
   E. narcotic drug overdose

131. A 42-year-old woman presents to Casualty with right-sided colicky loin pain and nausea for the past 3 hours. She cannot keep still because of the pain. She has a history of recurrent cystitis. Temperature 36.5°C, BP 110/60 and pulse 60/min. Urinalysis shows microscopic haematuria. The most likely diagnosis is:

   A. pelvic inflammatory disease
   B. acute pyelonephritis
   C. acute appendicitis
   D. renal colic
   E. ectopic pregnancy

132. The most useful initial diagnostic investigation is:

   A. serum urea and electrolytes
   B. urine βHCG
   C. plain KUB film
   D. pelvic ultrasound
   E. IV urogram

133. While in Casualty the patient develops fever and rigors. The most likely complication that has occurred is:

   A. ruptured ectopic pregnancy
   B. exacerbation of pelvic inflammatory disease
   C. ruptured appendix
   D. acute pyelonephritis
   E. septicaemia

134. A 16-year-old girl is brought to Casualty by her mother. She complains of persistent and worsening dull right-sided lower abdominal pain and spotting of blood per vagina. The mother insists her daughter is a virgin. On examination temperature 36.5°C, BP 90/50 and pulse 120/min. The lower abdomen is rigid with rebound tenderness in the right iliac fossa. Her period is overdue. The most appropriate management following resuscitation is:

A. Ask to speak to the girl in private, and obtain confidential information from her as to whether she has been sexually active. If so, perform a urinanalysis, urine βHCG pregnancy test and pelvic examination with triple swabs.
B. Arrange for urgent transvaginal ultrasound to exclude ectopic pregnancy.
C. Accept that the daughter is a virgin, omit a pelvic internal examination and take a low vaginal swab to exclude infection.
D. Arrange for pelvic ultrasound to exclude ectopic pregnancy and acute appendicitis.
E. Inform the mother that you are performing a urine pregnancy test in the best interests of her daughter to exclude possibility of a miscarriage or ectopic pregnancy.

135. A 70-year-old man presents to the outpatient clinic complaining of difficulty urinating and dribbling. On abdominal examination he has a distended bladder that reaches the umbilicus. He also complains of back pain. The NEXT most appropriate step would be:

A. take blood for serum urea, creatinine and electrolytes
B. take blood for PSA and acid phosphatase
C. perform a digital rectal examination
D. insert a Foley catheter
E. MSU for urinanalysis and MC&S

136. A 40-year-old woman presents with dysuria and urinary incontinence. She has a history of having passed urinary calculi in the past. The urine is noted to have an alkaline pH. The most likely organism is:

A. *Escherichia coli*
B. *Proteus mirabilis*
C. Atypical streptococci
D. *Pseudomonas aeruginosa*
E. *Klebsiella* sp.

137. A 40-year-old pedestrian has been struck by a speeding car. He is brought to Casualty wearing a pneumatic anti-shock garment for an extensive open avulsion injury to his pelvis. He is intubated with fluids running via two large-bore intra-venous cannulas. Blood pressure is 120/80. The pelvis is grossly distorted. The next most appropriate management as a casualty officer would be:

    A. take blood for FBC, type and cross 6 units, urea and electrolytes and commence O negative blood infusion
    B. cut away the man's clothing and perform a thorough physical examination
    C. insert a Foley catheter after a digital rectal examination to exclude a high-riding prostate
    D. perform a brief neurological examination
    E. notify the orthopaedic surgeons to apply an external fixator

138. An 18-year-old man presents with fever, stridor and trismus. His breathing becomes laboured with use of accessory muscles. He becomes cyanosed with a respiratory rate of 35, despite oxygen by face mask. He had initially presented to his GP a few days ago with a sore throat. He takes salbutamol inhaler for his asthma. The most appropriate management in Casualty would be:

    A. endotracheal intubation
    B. needle cricothyroidotomy
    C. tracheostomy
    D. IV hydrocortisone
    E. nasopharyngeal airway

139. The most likely diagnosis is:

    A. glandular fever
    B. streptococcal throat infection
    C. acute asthma attack
    D. angioneurotic oedema
    E. tetanus

140. A 60-year-old woman presents with progressive forgetfulness and mood changes. She has a shuffling gait. Her brain CT scan shows cortical atrophy and enlarged ventricles. Histology shows senile plaques and neurofibrillary tangles. The most appropriate treatment is:

A. levodopa in combination with a dopa-decarboxylase inhibitor
B. donepezil
C. tetrabenazine
D. diazepam
E. thiamine

141. The following statements regarding good medical practice are correct EXCEPT:

A. You may end professional relationships with patients if they have persistently acted inconsiderately.
B. You must assist the coroner by offering all relevant information to an inquest.
C. You are not entitled to remain silent if your evidence may lead to criminal proceedings being taken against you.
D. If you have grounds to believe that a doctor may be putting patients at risk, you must give an honest explanation of your concerns to a medical director.
E. You must not refuse to treat a patient because you may be putting yourself at risk.

142. A 60-year-old priest presents with cough, dyspnoea, dull chest pain and vague epigastric pain. On examination the left chest shows diminished expansion, stony dull percussion note and absent breath sounds. There is aegophony at the apex. The mediastium is shifted to the right. The chest x-ray confirms a unilateral pleural effusion. The most useful investigation would be:

A. CT chest
B. sputum for culture and sensitivity
C. aspiration of pleural effusion
D. bronchoscopy
E. V/Q scan

143. A 60-year-old man presents with increasing abdominal girth. On examination you elicit shifting dullness. The most useful investigation would be:

    A. CT scan of the abdomen
    B. ascitic fluid tap
    C. ultrasound of the abdomen
    D. chest x-ray
    E. blood for FBC, urea and electrolytes, LFTs and amylase

144. A 45-year-old woman presents with severe itching, recent pale stools and dark urine. On examination there is darkened skin pigmentation, xanthelasma and hepatomegaly. Test results are as follows:

    | serum bilirubin | 15 μmol/L |
    | serum alkaline phosphatase | 400 IU/L (30–300 IU/L) |
    | AST | 40 IU/L (5–35 IU/L) |

    The most likely diagnosis is:

    A. sarcoidosis
    B. primary biliary cirrhosis
    C. sclerosing cholangitis
    D. acute cholecystitis
    E. common bile duct gallstones

145. *Neisseria gonorrhoea* may infect all of the following areas EXCEPT:

    A. vagina
    B. rectum
    C. pharynx
    D. conjunctiva
    E. urethra

146. A 30-year-old woman with Crohn's disease presents with left flank pain and microscopic haematuria. She admits she doesn't drink enough water. She smokes, drinks wine and loves chocolates. X-ray shows a radio-opaque left renal calculus. The most likely aetiology is:

    A. hypercalciuria
    B. hyperoxaluria
    C. hyperuricaemia
    D. cystinuria
    E. hyperuricosuria

147. Dietary recommendations you would make for her include avoidance of all of the following EXCEPT:

A. spinach
B. rhubarb
C. chocolate
D. tomatoes
E. tea

148. A 50-year-old man with known liver disease presents with fever, abdominal pain and distension. On examination he has a tender abdomen with shifting dullness. Diagnostic aspiration shows elevated neutrophils. Gram stain shows Gram-negative rods. The most likely organism is:

A. *Klebsiella* sp.
B. *Escherichia coli*
C. *Pseudomonas aeruginosa*
D. *Bacteroides fragilis*
E. *Streptococcus pneumoniae*

149. Causes of air under the diaphragm include all of the following EXCEPT:

A. Crohn's disease
B. perforated duodenal ulcer
C. pleuroperitoneal fistula
D. laparoscopy
E. ruptured ectopic pregnancy

150. A 30-year-old man presents with fever, arthralgia and a palmar rash. On examination he has oral vesicles and target-like lesions on his palms. The most likely diagnosis is:

A. Stevens–Johnson syndrome
B. Behçet's syndrome
C. herpes simplex
D. syphilis
E. hand-foot-mouth disease

151. A 50-year-old man presents in shock with rigors and a temperature of 40°C. He is jaundiced and is tender on palpation of the liver, which is felt 5 cm below the costal margin. Dark concentrated urine is noted upon Foley catheter insertion. The most likely diagnosis is:

A. ascending cholangitis
B. gallstone ileus
C. hepatitis
D. primary sclerosing cholangitis
E. acute cholecystitis

152. A 60-year-old woman presents with morning stiffness in both knees and pain worse at the end of the day. On examination the knees are swollen and warm to the touch. She has a flexion deformity and limitation of movement. X-ray shows narrowing of the joint spaces, osteophytes at the margin of the joints and sclerosis of the underlying bone. The most likely diagnosis is:

A. rheumatoid arthritis
B. osteoarthritis
C. gout
D. infective arthritis
E. polymyalgia rheumatica

153. Recognised treatments for this condition include all of the following EXCEPT:

A. total knee replacement
B. NSAIDs
C. penicillamine
D. intra-articular corticosteroid
E. physiotherapy

154. A 70-year-old man presents with progressive stepwise dementia associated with focal neurological events. He has a stiff, slow-moving, spastic tongue, dysarthria and inappropriate laughing and crying. He walks with a shuffling gait taking small steps. He is also noted to be hypertensive. The most likely diagnosis is:

A. Parkinson's disease
B. Alzheimer's disease
C. multi-infarct dementia
D. lateral medullary syndrome
E. multiple sclerosis

155. A 20-year-old man complains of recurrent lower back pain and stiffness after exercise. He has no morning stiffness. Full blood count and ESR are normal, but he is found to have HLA-B27. X-ray of his lumbar spine and pelvis are normal. The most appropriate management would be:

    A. no further investigations and reassure the patient that HLA-B27 can also be found in normal people
    B. arrange for an ophthamology referral for slit-lamp examination
    C. arrange a Kveim test to exclude sarcoidosis
    D. arrange for barium follow-through
    E. test for rheumatoid factor

156. A 55-year-old insulin-dependent diabetic presents with nausea, lethargy, dry and itchy yellow-brown skin. He also complains of nocturia and impotence. His blood film shows normocytic normochromic anaemia and occasional Burr cells. The most appropriate management would be:

    A. commence iron replacement therapy
    B. take blood for urea and electrolytes
    C. check HbAIC
    D. take blood for bilirubin, LFTs and amylase
    E. take blood for thyroid function tests

157. Cystic fibrosis is associated with all of the following EXCEPT:

    A. abnormal gene coding for transmembrane regulating factor protein on chromosome 7
    B. allergic bronchopulmonary aspergillosis
    C. steatorrhoea
    D. chronic infection with *Pseudomonas pseudomallei*
    E. diabetes mellitus

158. A 20-year-old pregnant black woman presents with fever and joint pains. She has a history of two previous spontaneous early miscarriages. Urine reveals 2+ protein. Blood results show leucopenia, normocytic normochromic anaemia and thrombocytopenia. The most likely diagnosis is:

    A. sickle-cell disease
    B. SLE
    C. thalassaemia
    D. aplastic anaemia
    E. pre-eclampsia

159. The most sensitive diagnostic test would be:

    A. PET screen
    B. antibodies to double-stranded DNA
    C. positive anti-nuclear antibodies
    D. antibody to Ro
    E. haemoglobin electrophoresis

160. The most useful investigation for her miscarriages would be:

    A. transvaginal ultrasound
    B. chromosome karyotype
    C. lupus anticoagulant and anticardiolipin antibody
    D. hysterosalpingogram
    E. antithrombin III, protein C and S deficiency

161. The most common organism implicated in acute bacterial endocarditis is:

    A. *Staphylococcus aureus*
    B. *Streptococcus viridans*
    C. *Streptococcus faecalis*
    D. *Staphylococcus epidermidis*
    E. *Coxiella burneti*

162. A 25-year-old heroin addict presents with fever and mucosal petechial haemorrhages. On examination he has a pansystolic murmur best heard at the lower sternal edge. He is also noted to have small, flat, erythematous, non-tender macules over the thenar eminence. The most likely diagnosis is:

    A. subacute bacterial endocarditis
    B. acute bacterial endocarditis
    C. rheumatic heart disease
    D. acute rheumatic fever
    E. Q fever

163. Major criteria for the diagnosis of rheumatic fever include all of the following EXCEPT:

    A. polyarthralgia
    B. chorea
    C. erythema marginatum
    D. subcutaneous nodules
    E. fever

164. The organism responsible for gas gangrene is:

   A. *Clostridium difficile*
   B. *Clostridium perfringens*
   C. *Clostridium tetani*
   D. *Klebsiella* sp.
   E. *Pseudomonas aeruginosa*

165. Which one of the following features would favour a diagnosis of Guillain–Barré syndrome rather than myasthenia gravis?

   A. ocular muscle involvement
   B. proximal muscle weakness
   C. respiratory difficulties
   D. areflexia
   E. facial muscle weakness

166. The most common cause of painless frank haematuria in male patients over 50 years old is:

   A. bladder squamous cell carcinoma
   B. carcinoma of the prostate
   C. hypernephroma
   D. transitional cell carcinoma in the kidney
   E. transitional cell bladder carcinoma

167. A 30-year-old man presents to Casualty with a tender swollen testicle. He states that he was struck in the groin while playing football. On examination the borders of the testicle are irregular, and the testicle is heavy and woody. There is no associated lymphadenopathy. He is also noted to have gynaecomastia. There are no external signs of trauma. The most appropriate initial management would be:

   A. take blood for α-fetoprotein and βHCG and arrange for a chest x-ray
   B. prescribe doxycycline 100 mg o bd for 5 days
   C. refer to urologists for urgent surgical exploration
   D. arrange for a chest and abdominal CT scan
   E. arrange for an ultrasound of the testes

168. A 20-year-old female presents with acne and hirsutism. She complains of a year of chaotic menstrual cycles with long periods of amenorrhoea. She has gained weight recently. She has never been pregnant. On examination there are no other abnormalities. The most likely diagnosis is:

   A. congenital adrenal hyperplasia
   B. ovarian teratoma
   C. Cushing's disease
   D. testicular feminisation
   E. polycystic ovarian disease

169. Treatment for multiple sclerosis includes all of the following EXCEPT:

   A. glatiramer actetate
   B. interferon beta-1a
   C. interferon beta-1b
   D. interferon alfa
   E. baclofen

170. Which one of the following features would favour a diagnosis of ulcerative colitis rather than Crohn's disease?

   A. uveitis
   B. arthritis
   C. pyoderma gangrenosum
   D. cholelithiasis
   E. pseudopolyps

171. A 50-year-old man presents with polydipsia, headache and weakness. On examination BP is 160/100 but he is not oedematous. He takes no medication. Blood results reveal hypokalaemia, alkalosis and low serum renin. The most likely diagnosis is:

   A. Conn's syndrome
   B. secondary hyperaldosteronism
   C. Cushing's disease
   D. phaeochromocytoma
   E. renal artery stenosis

172. A 25-year-old healthy male smoker presents with gangrene of the left big toe. There are no signs of external trauma. The most likely diagnosis is:

    A. thrombangiitis obliterans (Buerger's disease)
    B. Raynaud's disease
    C. gas gangrene
    D. polyarteritis nodosa
    E. gout

173. Peptic ulcer disease is associated with all of the following EXCEPT:

    A. head trauma
    B. burns
    C. chronic pancreatitis
    D. hypocalcaemia
    E. cirrhosis

174. The most common cause of massive upper gastrointestinal bleeding is:

    A. gastric ulcer
    B. duodenal ulcer
    C. oesophageal varices
    D. Mallory–Weiss syndrome
    E. angiodysplasia

175. A 35-year-old African woman is found to have a Hb of 6 g/dL. She is a vegetarian and has a history of uterine fibroids. Blood film reveals microcytic, hypochromic red blood cells and a few target cells. The most likely result of iron studies would be:

    A. low ferritin, high TIBC
    B. low iron, low TIBC
    C. raised ferritin, low TIBC
    D. low serum iron, low TIBC
    E. normal ferritin, high TIBC

176. A 40-year-old long-stay patient in a psychiatric hospital presents with fever, abdominal pain, dry cough and worsening confusion. Blood tests reveal neutrophilia, lymphopenia and hyponatraemia. Chest x-ray shows right-sided lobar consolidation. The most appropriate treatment would be:

    A. erythromycin
    B. benzylpenicillin
    C. antituberculous chemotherapy
    D. ciprofloxacin
    E. ticarcillin

177. Diseases associated with impotence include all of the following EXCEPT:

    A. hypothyroidism
    B. hyperprolactinaemia
    C. cirrhosis
    D. multiple sclerosis
    E. renal failure

178. The following are symptoms of schizophrenia EXCEPT:

    A. obsessional intrusive thoughts
    B. thought insertion
    C. poverty of speech
    D. suspiciousness
    E. primary delusion

179. A 20-year-old man who has travelled recently to India presents with unexplained fever for 5 days. You suspect typhoid fever. The most appropriate investigation would be:

    A. Widal test measuring serum levels of agglutinins to O and H antigens
    B. blood culture
    C. marrow culture
    D. stool culture
    E. urine culture

180. The following statements regarding sarcoidosis are correct EXCEPT:

    A. There is a higher incidence among young black males than caucasians
    B. It most commonly involves the mediastinal lymph nodes
    C. A third of cases are associated with erythema nodosum
    D. Scalene node biopsy will be positive in 90% of cases
    E. A negative Kveim test excludes sarcoidosis.

181. A 70-year-old man presents with chronic cough, haemoptysis and weight loss. He smokes 20 cigarettes a day. Chest x-ray shows a central coin lesion. The most useful investigation would be:

    A. sputum for culture and cytology
    B. isotope bone scan
    C. bronchoscopy and biopsy
    D. percutaneous needle biopsy
    E. chest CT scan

182. Pelvic inflammatory disease is associated with all of the following EXCEPT:

    A. infertility
    B. ectopic pregnancies
    C. Chlamydia trachomatis infection
    D. tubo-ovarian abscess
    E. endometriosis

183. The most common viral illness in transplant patients is:

    A. human immunodeficiency virus
    B. herpes zoster
    C. herpes simplex
    D. cytomegalovirus
    E. Ebstein–Barr virus

184. A 30-year-old woman presents with a diffusely enlarged thyroid gland associated with a bruit. Serum thyroxine is raised and TSH is low. The most discriminating investigation would be:

A. ultrasound scan
B. fine-needle biopsy
C. serum thyroid-stimulating immunoglobulins against TSH receptor
D. radioiodine scan
E. thyroid releasing hormone (TRH) test

185. A 50-year-old woman is noted to have a high serum calcium, low-normal phosphate and normal albumin on routine biochemistry test. She is asymptomatic. The most useful additional blood test would be:

A. serum chloride
B. serum parathyroid hormone (PTH)
C. serum magnesium
D. serum urea
E. serum alkaline phosphatase

186. The serum parathyroid hormone (PTH) comes back as high. The most useful investigation to confirm the diagnosis is:

A. skull x-ray
B. pelvic x-ray
C. radioisotope thallium/technetium subtraction scan of the neck
D. chest x-ray
E. CT scan of the neck

187. A 90-year-old man is noted to have a serum alkaline phosphatase of 1050 IU/L (30–300 IU/L) on routine blood tests. He is asymptomatic. Serum calcium, phosphate, and PTH levels are normal. The most likely diagnosis is:

A. multiple myeloma
B. osteitis deformans
C. bone metastases
D. hyperparathyroidism
E. osteomalacia

188. A 20-year-old man back from hitchhiking through South America a fortnight ago now presents with explosive watery foul-smelling diarrhoea and weight loss. On examination he has abdominal distension. His stools are greasy and contain mucus. The most useful investigation would be:

    A. proctoscopy
    B. sodium sweat test
    C. abdominal x-ray
    D. stool for microscopy
    E. duodenal aspirate

189. A 60-year-old man collapses on the ward. ECG shows asystole. There is no palpable carotid pulse. The most appropriate management is:

    A. DC cardioversion starting at 200 J
    B. 1 minute of CPR during which the airway is secured and 1 mg of epinephrine (adrenaline) IV is administered
    C. 3 minutes of CPR during which the airway is secured and 3 mg of atropine IV is administered
    D. repeated precordial blows at a rate of 70/min (percussion pacing)
    E. 3 minutes of CPR during which the airway is secured and both epinephrine (adrenaline) and atropine IV are administered

190. A 30-year-old man presents in coma following drug overdose. His pupils are dilated, and he is hypotensive. His pulse rate drops to 40 and ECG confirms second degree Mobitz type II heart block. The most likely cause of his overdose is:

    A. barbiturate
    B. tricyclic antidepressant
    C. lithium
    D. beta-blocker
    E. benzodiazepine

191. A 50-year-old obese man presents with headache and drowsiness. He has a history of snoring. He has warm extremities, a flapping tremor and a bounding pulse. On fundoscopic examination papilloedema is present. The most likely cause for the papilloedema is:

    A. CO_2 retention
    B. hypoxia
    C. obstructive sleep apnoea
    D. cerebral tumour
    E. malignant hypertension

192. A 25-year-old woman presents to casualty with light-headedness and breathlessness. She complains of tingling and numbness of her hands. Arterial blood gas:

pH	7.55
Pa_{CO_2}	3 kPa
Pa_{O_2}	14 kPa
H^+	25 nmol/L
HCO_3	20 mmol/L

The most appropriate management would be:

A. chest x-ray
B. breathe into a paper bag
C. activated charcoal
D. needle thoracentesis
E. V/Q scan

193. A 20-year-old asthmatic presents with increased shortness of breath. On chest examination he is found to have a deviated trachea to the right, reduced tactile fremitus and hyperresonance to percussion on the left. The most likely diagnosis is:

A. right-sided pulmonary embolism
B. right-sided pneumothorax
C. left-sided pneumothorax
D. left bronchopneumonia
E. left-sided pleural effusion

194. A 50-year-old man presents with weight loss, hiccoughs, jaundice, epigastric and right upper quadrant pain radiating to the back. On examination he is noted to have hepatomegaly, a palpable gallbladder and an abdominal bruit heard in the periumbilical area and left upper quadrant. The most likely diagnosis is:

A. abdominal aortic aneurysm
B. gallbladder carcinoma
C. hepatocellular carcinoma
D. carcinoma of the head of the pancreas
E. cholecystitis

195. Recognised side-effects of thiazide diuretics include all of the following EXCEPT:

    A. hyperuricaemia
    B. increased LDL cholesterol
    C. hypokalaemia
    D. hypoglycaemia
    E. hypercalcaemia

196. First-line therapy for hypertension in a pregnant woman is:

    A. atenolol
    B. hydralazine
    C. methyldopa
    D. bendrofluazide
    E. nifedipine

197. A 50-year-old man with IDDM presents with peripheral oedema and ascites. He has 3+ proteinuria. 24-hour urine collection contains 10 g of protein. Serum albumin is 15 g/L. The most likely diagnosis is:

    A. diabetic nephrosclerosis
    B. nephrotic syndrome
    C. uraemia
    D. interstitial nephritis
    E. retroperitoneal fibrosis

198. A 25-year-old HIV-positive man presents with two weeks of worsening drowsiness. On examination he has cervical lymphadenopathy and has bilateral upgoing plantar reflexes. CT scan of the head shows cerebral calcifications and ring lesions. The most likely diagnosis is:

    A. cerebral toxoplasmosis
    B. cerebral abscess
    C. lymphoma
    D. cryptococcus meningitis
    E. tuberculosis

199. A 12-year-old boy presents to Casualty with severe dyspnoea. He had been treated by his GP with penicillin for presumed tonsillitis. He uses a salbutamol inhaler for asthma. On examination: temperature 40°C and he is drooling saliva; no trismus. Marked inspiratory stridor and a respiratory rate of 30/min. The most appropriate management would be:

   A. oxygen-driven nebuliser
   B. IV hydrocortisone
   C. indirect laryngoscopy
   D. endotracheal intubation under general anaesthesia
   E. cricothyroidotomy

200. The most likely diagnosis is:

   A. croup
   B. acute epiglottitis
   C. glandular fever
   D. acute streptococcal tonsillitis
   E. acute severe asthma attack

201. A 50-year-old man with a history of previous myocardial infarction presents to Casualty with chest pain. The initial blood pressure is 110/70. During evaluation, he collapses. ECG shows ventricular tachycardia. He has no palpable pulse. The most appropriate management would be:

   A. synchronised DC shock at 100 J
   B. administer IV amiodarone 150 mg over 10 minutes
   C. DC cardioversion with 200 J
   D. administer IV lidocaine (lignocaine) 50 mg over 2 minutes
   E. commence CPR

202. An 80-year-old woman presents with chronic dysphagia and weight loss. She complains of a sensation of a lump in her throat, bad breath and regurgitation of undigested food. She has a history of recurrent chest infections. She does not smoke or drink alcohol. Physical examination reveals a low BMI and a visible lump on the left side of her neck, which is difficult to define on palpation. The most definitive investigation would be:

   A. chest x-ray
   B. barium meal
   C. endoscopy and biopsy
   D. oesophageal motility studies
   E. indirect laryngoscopy

203. A 30-year-old woman presents with bilateral ptosis and diplopia. She has also noticed difficulty in swallowing. The most likely diagnosis is:

A. dystrophia myotonica
B. multiple sclerosis
C. polymyositis
D. myasthenic syndrome (Eaton–Lambert syndrome)
E. myasthenia gravis

204. A 20-year-old woman presents with complete right ptosis. On lifting the eyelid, the eye is seen to be looking down and out. The pupil is dilated. The most likely diagnosis is:

A. right third nerve and right superior oblique palsy
B. complete right third nerve palsy
C. incomplete right third nerve palsy
D. Horner's syndrome
E. right third nerve and lateral rectus palsy

205. The following conditions can mimic panic disorder EXCEPT:

A. phaeochromocytoma
B. hyperthyroidism
C. hypoglycaemia
D. caffeine withdrawal
E. barbiturate withdrawal

206. A 20-year-old man presents for psychotherapy. He is manipulative and lacks empathy. He has a grandiose sense of self-importance and entitlement. The most likely personality disorder would be described as:

A. antisocial
B. borderline
C. histrionic
D. schizotypal
E. narcissistic

207. A 22-year-old female presents with secondary amenorrhoea and weight loss. On examination she is noted to have mild parotid swelling. She has a low BP and a BMI of 15. The most likely reason for her amenorrhoea is:

A. prolactinoma
B. Addison's disease
C. premature ovarian failure
D. anorexia nervosa
E. bulimia

208. The treatment of choice for adolescent-onset Gilles de la Tourette's syndrome is:

A. ritalin
B. pimozide
C. haloperidol
D. clonidine
E. clonazepam

209. The most common cause of new-onset focal or generalised seizures after the age of 50 is:

A. alcoholism
B. brain abscess
C. brain tumour
D. cerebrovascular disease
E. encephalitis

210. An 80-year-old man presents with a 2-month history of weakness, dark stools and worsening constipation alternating with episodes of diarrhoea. He has lost a stone in weight. He has a history of diverticular disease and has had two myocardial infarctions. Blood tests reveal anaemia, hyponatraemia, hypokalaemia and hypochloraemia. The stool is positive for occult blood. The most useful diagnostic investigation is:

A. chest and abdominal plain x-rays
B. mesenteric angiography
C. barium enema
D. sigmoidoscopy
E. barium swallow and meal

211. A 15-year-old boy presents with high swinging fever and arthritis affecting the knees. The joints are swollen but not very tender. Blood tests reveal anaemia and a raised ESR. Rheumatoid factor is negative but anti-nuclear antibodies are positive. The most likely diagnosis is:

A. acute rheumatic fever
B. juvenile rheumatoid arthritis
C. Still's disease
D. osteochondritis dissecans
E. aseptic non-traumatic synovitis

212. The next most appropriate step to guide your further management would be:

A. echocardiography
B. aspiration of knee joint
C. arrange for MRI scan of the knee
D. arrange for ophthalmology referral for slit-lamp examination
E. blood cultures

213. A 30-year-old man presents with acute loin pain and haematuria. He has a history of recurrent urinary tract infections. He states that his father also had kidney problems and had suffered from a bleed in the brain. On examination BP is 160/100, and he has ballotable large, irregular kidneys and hepatomegaly. The most definitive investigation would be:

A. kidney-ureter-bladder plain film
B. excretion urography
C. CT scan of the abdomen
D. renal ultrasound
E. urinalysis and MSU for culture and sensitivities

214. The following are first-rank symptoms of schizophrenia EXCEPT:

A. anhedonia
B. bodily sensations being imposed by an outside agency
C. delusional perceptions
D. third person auditory hallucinations
E. alien thoughts

215. Postsplenectomy complications include all of the following EXCEPT:

A. falciparum malaria
B. *Haemophilus influenzae* infection
C. pneumococcal septicaemia
D. thromboembolism
E. thrombocytopenia

216. A 60-year-old man with a history of angina presents with chest pain. ECG shows ventricular tachycardia. Pulse rate is 200/min, and BP 80/50. Oxygen is applied by face mask. Initial management should be:

A. administer sedation and call urgently for the anaesthetist
B. immediate synchronised cardioversion at 100 J
C. immediate unsynchronised DC cardioversion at 200 J
D. IV adenosine
E. IV lidocaine (lignocaine)

217. A 20-year-old man complains of high fever, rigors, productive cough with rusty-coloured sputum and pleuritic chest pain. On chest examination he has increased tactile fremitus and dullness to percussion in the right lower lung field. The most likely diagnosis is:

A. lobar pneumonia
B. bronchopneumonia
C. aspiration pneumonia
D. pleural effusion
E. lung abscess

218. A 40-year-old woman presents with multiple symptoms. She states that for weeks she has felt tired with a loss of appetite. She has intermittent abdominal pain, diarrhoea and has lost half a stone in weight. On examination: temperature 36.5°C, supine BP 100/60 with a pulse of 90/min; postural hypotension, mild epigastric pain and a pigmented appendicectomy scar. The most likely diagnosis is:

A. hypopituitarism
B. diabetes mellitus
C. Addison's disease
D. hyperthyroidism
E. Crohn's syndrome

219. A 25-year-old obese lady presents with mood swings, acne, secondary amenorrhoea and hirsutism. She has mild lower back pain, which she relates to her weight problem. She smokes 20 cigarettes a day and drinks alcohol on weekends. BP is 125/85 and urine dipstick is negative for glucose. The most likely diagnosis is:

A. Cushing's syndrome
B. polycystic ovary syndrome
C. congenital adrenal hyperplasia
D. ovarian carcinoma
E. hypothyroidism

220. A 90-year-old man is noted to have a serum alkaline phosphatase of 1050 IU/L (30–300 IU/L) on routine blood tests. He is asymptomatic. Serum calcium, phosphate and PTH levels are normal. The most appropriate treatment would be:

A. nil
B. parathyroid surgeon referral
C. chest x-ray
D. vitamin D therapy
E. calcitonin

221. A 50-year-old obese man is brought to Casualty in a confused state. On examination he has nystagmus and is unable to move the eyes fully laterally. He walks with a broad-based gait. He is unaware of his surroundings and grows restless. The most likely diagnosis is:

A. subdural haematoma
B. Creutzfeldt–Jakob syndrome
C. Wernicke's encephalopathy
D. Korsakoff's psychosis
E. hypoglycaemia

222. A 60-year-old woman with rheumatoid arthritis presents with neck pain and numbness and tingling in the thumb and first two fingers of the right hand. It is worse at night. On examination there is sensory loss in the right hand involving the lateral half of the ring finger and dorsal tips of the first two fingers. The patient is able to flex the interphalangeal joint of the index finger on clasping the hands (Ochner's test). The most likely diagnosis is:

A. complete median nerve lesion
B. carpal tunnel syndrome
C. median and ulnar nerve palsy
D. cervical spondylosis
E. cervical rib

223. The most useful investigation is:

A. lateral and antero-posterior cervical-spine x-ray
B. MRI scan of the neck
C. nerve conduction studies
D. hand x-ray
E. chest x-ray

224. A 40-year-old man presents with diplopia and pain over the left eye. His medication includes lisinopril and Humulin insulin. On examination he has an almost total ophthalmoplegia with sparing of lateral eye movement on the left. His pupils are symmetrical, reactive to light and are of normal size and shape. The most likely diagnosis is:

A. III nerve palsy due to compression
B. mononeuritis involving the III nerve
C. complete III nerve palsy
D. Argyll Robertson pupil
E. myasthenia gravis

225. A 30-year-old female presents with severe headache and vomiting. She is sensitive to light and also complains of neck pain. BP is 170/110 and pulse 50. On examination she has bilateral ptosis, dilated pupils and eyes are positioned down and out. On fundoscopic examination bilateral papilloedema is present. Protein and glucose are present in her urine. Her mental status deteriorates rapidly. The most likely diagnosis is:

A. intracranial tumour
B. subdural haematoma
C. subarachnoid haemorrhage
D. extradural haematoma
E. intracerebral haemorrhage

226. The most appropriate investigation is:

A. lumbar puncture
B. head CT scan
C. MRI scan of the brain
D. cerebral angiography
E. electroencephalogram

227. A 50-year-old woman complains of episodes of diplopia and vertigo, worse after exercise. On examination the BP in her right arm is 120/80 and the BP in her left arm is 100/60. A cervical bruit is noted. The most likely diagnosis is:

A. coarctation of the aorta
B. transient ischaemic attack
C. Takayasu's arteritis
D. subclavian steal syndrome
E. vertebrobasilar insufficiency

228. A 50-year-old obese man presents with headache and drowsiness. He has a history of snoring. He has warm extremities, a flapping tremor and a bounding pulse. On fundoscopic examination papilloedema is present. The most appropriate treatment would be:

A. flumazenil
B. doxapram
C. naloxone
D. hyperbaric oxygen
E. diazepam

229. A 70-year-old man presents with nausea, vomiting and weakness. He has marked peripheral oedema. His medications include digoxin and chlorthalidone for congestive heart failure. Frusemide is administered to which he has marked diuresis of 10 litres and promptly collapses. ECG shows prolonged P-R interval, inverted T waves and depressed ST segments. The most useful blood test is:

A. CK-MB and troponin
B. serum urea and electrolytes
C. digoxin level
D. serum osmolality
E. random cortisol

230. A 40-year-old man presents with painful asymmetrical deforming arthritis involving the distal interphalangeal joints and lower back pain. His fingernails are pitted, with onycholysis and linear melanonychia. The most likely diagnosis is:

A. rheumatoid arthritis
B. ankylosing spondylitis
C. psoriatic arthritis
D. osteoarthritis
E. ulcerative colitis

231. A 16-year-old male presents with gynaecomastia. On examination his arm span exceeds the body length and he has small, firm testes. The most likely diagnosis is:

A. testicular feminisation
B. congenital adrenal hyperplasia
C. Klinefelter's syndrome
D. true hermaphroditism
E. adrenal 5α-reductase deficiency

232. A 45-year-old female who underwent mastectomy with axillary clearance 2 years ago now presents with excessive thirst and polyuria. Investigations show:

serum sodium	150 mmol/L
serum potassium	3.8 mmol/L
serum calcium	2.8 mmol/L
random serum glucose	9 mmol/L
serum urea	6 mmol/L
serum creatinine	100 µmol/L
urine osmolality	150 mosm/L

The most likely diagnosis is:

A. psychogenic polydipsia
B. SIADH
C. diabetes insipidus
D. hypercalcaemia
E. diabetes mellitus

233. A 65-year-old woman presents to Casualty with breathlessness and chest pain. On examination the pulse is irregularly irregular and ECG confirms atrial fibrillation at a rate of 180/min. You administer oxygen and gain IV access. The next most appropriate step in management would be:

A. heparin and warfarin anticoagulation
B. immediate heparin and synchronised DC shock at 100 J
C. amiodarone 300 mg IV over 1 hour
D. IV digoxin
E. flecainide 100 mg IV over 30 minutes

234. A 22-year-old female presents with frothy grey vaginal discharge. She states that she last had unprotected sexual intercourse 2 weeks ago. The vaginal discharge emits a fishy odour on alkalinisation with potassium hydroxide and is noted to have a pH of 5. The most likely organism is:

A. *Neisseria gonorrhoea*
B. *Trichomonas vaginalis*
C. candidiasis
D. *Chlamydia trachomatis*
E. *Gardnerella vaginalis*

235. An 80-year-old woman presents with chronic dysphagia and weight loss. She complains of a sensation of a lump in her throat, bad breath, and regurgitation of undigested food. She has a history of recurrent chest infections. She does not smoke or drink alcohol. Physical examination reveals a low BMI and a visible lump on the left side of her neck, which is difficult to define on palpation. The most likely diagnosis is:

A. squamous cell carcinoma of the oesophagus
B. pharyngeal pouch
C. achalasia
D. cricopharyngeal spasm
E. postcricoid carcinoma

236. A 60-year-old woman presents with sudden painless loss of vision in her right eye. There is no perception of light and there is an afferent pupillary defect. The retina is white with a cherry red spot at the macula. The optic discs are swollen. She also has a right-sided carotid bruit. The most likely diagnosis is:

A. retinal detachment
B. optic neuritis
C. central retinal vein occlusion
D. ischaemic optic neuropathy
E. central retinal artery occlusion

237. A 20-year-old woman presents with fatigue, nausea, vomiting, and abdominal colic. She has been feeling unwell for many months now and lives as a squatter in a derelict old house. On examination she is noted to have signs of peripheral neuropathy with a wrist drop. Blood film shows basophilic stippling of red blood cells. The most likely diagnosis is:

A. thalassaemia
B. iron poisoning
C. lead poisoning
D. Crohn's disease
E. carbon monoxide poisoning

238. A 28-year-old Jamaican woman presents with acute onset of nausea, vomiting, epigastric pain and ascites. She does not take any medication apart from traditional herbal remedies. On examination she has tender hepatomegaly and profound ascites but no signs of heart failure. She has abnormal LFTs. The ascitic fluid has high protein content. The investigation of choice is:

A. isotope scanning of the liver
B. hepatic venography
C. liver biopsy
D. ultrasound scan
E. abdominal x-ray

239. The most likely diagnosis is:

A. primary biliary cirrhosis
B. hepatic vein thrombosis
C. alcoholic hepatitis
D. portal vein thrombosis
E. Meig's syndrome

240. A 30-year-old HIV-positive male presents with seizures. The most likely infective cause is:

A. toxoplasmosis
B. cytomegalovirus
C. cryptosporidium
D. tuberculosis
E. pneumocystosis

241. Which of the following illicit drugs is still detectable in urine up to a month later?

A. cocaine
B. cannabis
C. methadone
D. heroin
E. amphetamine

242. A 50-year-old woman presents with an abdominal mass and back pain. She denies abdominal pain or abnormal vaginal bleeding having had her last period 9 months ago. Cervical smears have never been abnormal. On examination there is a central mass palpable to above the level of the umbilicus. On pelvic examination there is a palpable right adnexal mass. Urine HCG is negative. The most useful investigation is:

A. plain abdominal and lumbar spine x-rays
B. CT scan of the abdomen and pelvis
C. serum progesterone and β-HCG
D. pelvic ultrasound
E. CEA-125 tumour marker

243. A 50-year-old woman presents to medical outpatients complaining of pain and stiffness in the joints of her hands, worse in the mornings. The pain lasts for a couple of hours in the morning. On examination she has ulnar deviation, wasting of the small muscles of her hands, nail pitting and a rash on her knees. There is symmetrical involvement of the distal interphalangeal joints and metacarpophalangeal joints. The most likely diagnosis is:

A. rheumatoid arthritis
B. psoriatic arthropathy
C. Sjögren's syndrome
D. SLE
E. osteoarthritis

244. A 70-year-old man presents to Casualty after falling when drunk. He complains of sudden numbness and tingling all over both his legs. He also complains of pain between the shoulder blades. On examination he has weakness in his lower extremities, hyperreflexia, positive Babinski and clonus. The most likely diagnosis is:

A. motor neurone disease
B. subacute combined degeneration of the cord
C. spinal cord compression
D. cauda equina compression
E. anterior spinal artery occlusion

245. A 65-year-old man presents with a 2-month history of vague lower abdominal pain, alternating diarrhoea with constipation and 4 kg weight loss. He has passed a small amount of dark red blood per rectum. There is anaemia. The most likely diagnosis is:

A. diverticular disease
B. Crohn's disease
C. ulcerative colitis
D. angiodysplasia
E. carcinoma of the colon

246. The most useful investigation is:

A. flexible sigmoidoscopy
B. barium enema
C. CT scan of the abdomen
D. abdominal ultrasound
E. selective mesenteric angiography

247. A 35-year-old female presents with a 1-month history of a painless firm but mobile 2-cm lump in the upper outer quadrant of her breast. No other abnormalities detected. Initial investigation should be:

A. mammogram
B. ultrasound
C. fine needle aspiration cytology
D. trucut biopsy
E. assessment for BRCAI and 2 mutations with sentinel node biopsy

248. The most likely diagnosis is:

A. breast carcinoma
B. fibrocystic disease
C. fibroadenoma
D. benign mammary dysplasia
E. lipoma

249. A 60-year-old man presents to Casualty with fever and neck pain on passively moving the chin towards the chest. Lumbar puncture shows:

white cells	3000/cc predominantly neutrophils
red blood cells	1/cc
glucose	1.5 mmol/L
protein	5 g/L

The most likely organism is:

A. *Mycobacterium tuberculosis*
B. *Neisseria meningitidis*
C. *Haemophilus influenzae*
D. *Listeria monocytogenes*
E. *Streptococcus pneumoniae*

250. A 20-year-old female is referred for recurrent epistaxis and bruising. She takes no medication. On examination she has no facial rash or lymphadenopathy. Her spleen is mildly enlarged, and she has generalised bruising but no bone or joint tenderness. Immediate blood test results are:

white cell count	5×10^9/L
Hb	10 g/dL
platelets	25×10^9/L
ESR	55 mm/h
MCV	90 fl
MCH	30 pg
MCHC	34 g/dL
prolonged bleeding time	
serum urea	6 mmol/L

The next most useful investigation would be:

A. bone marrow aspirate
B. haemoglobin electrophoresis
C. platelet autoantibodies
D. Factor VIII : C and Factor VIII : vWF assays
E. platelet aggregation studies

251. The most likely diagnosis is:

A. thrombotic thrombocytopenic purpura
B. idiopathic thrombocytopenic purpura
C. aplastic anaemia
D. SLE
E. von Willebrand's disease

252. A 70-year-old man presents with confusion and urinary incontinence. He is pale; BP 160/100. On examination the bladder is palpable to the level of the umbilicus. Rectal examination confirms an enlarged prostate. There is also peripheral oedema. Blood tests show:

white cell count	7×10^9/L
Hb	8 g/dL
platelets	100×10^9/L
serum sodium	125 mmol/L
serum potassium	6 mmol/L
serum urea	60 mmol/L
serum calcium	3.4 mmol/L

The diagnosis is:

A. chronic renal failure
B. acute renal failure
C. benign prostatic hypertrophy
D. prostate carcinoma
E. myelomatosis

253. The most appropriate management would be:

A. arrange urgent renal ultrasound
B. slow bladder decompression with a sterile catheter
C. measure 24 hour urinary protein and creatinine clearance
D. arrange urgent IV urogram
E. give 10 ml of 10% calcium gluconate and 15 units of insulin with 50 g glucose 50% IV

254. A 22-year-old female is noted to have both microcyctic and macrocytic anaemia. She gives a history of intermittent diarrhoea with difficulty in flushing the stools. The most likely diagnosis is:

A. cystic fibrosis
B. irritable bowel syndrome
C. coeliac disease
D. Crohn's disease
E. ulcerative colitis

255. A 60-year-old man presents with sudden severe colicky pain and bloody diarrhoea that began after lunch 3 hours ago. He has a history of two myocardial infarctions. On examination: temperature 39°C, BP 130/90, pulse 110/min regular. There is rebound tenderness in the lower left quadrant of his abdomen and there is fresh blood present in the rectum. There is a raised white cell count and mild anaemia. The most likely diagnosis is:

A. colon carcinoma
B. diverticular disease
C. inferior mesenteric artery ischaemia
D. superior mesenteric artery thromboembolism
E. campylobacter infection

256. A 20-year-old man presents with morning back stiffness. He has a history of iritis. On examination he has an early-diastolic murmur. Chest x-ray shows bilateral diffuse reticulonodular shadowing. The most likely diagnosis is:

A. Reiter's syndrome
B. Crohn's disease
C. rheumatoid arthritis
D. ankylosing spondylitis
E. sacro-iliitis

257. An asymptomatic 60-year-old man is found to have an isolated raised alkaline phosphatase on routine biochemistry. Serum calcium and phosphate levels are normal. The most likely diagnosis is:

A. osteomalacia
B. multiple myeloma
C. Paget's disease
D. cirrhosis
E. hyperparathyroidism

258. The most suitable treatment for *Clostridium difficile* is:

A. vancomycin
B. amoxicillin
C. gentamicin
D. cimetidine
E. tetracycline

259. What would be the most suitable laxative to offer a termi-
nally ill patient hooked up to a morphine syringe driver?

A. lactulose
B. co-danthromer
C. loperamide
D. methylcellulose
E. phosphate enema

260. A 50-year-old man with IDDM is commenced on enalapril
for hypertension. Two weeks later his U+Es results are noted
to be abnormal. What is the most likely cause?

A. renal papillary necrosis
B. hypovolaemia
C. Addison's disease
D. renal artery stenosis
E. renal tumour

261. A dockyard worker is referred to the chest clinic for breathlessness. Chest x-ray shows pleural thickening and calcification (pleural plaques). What is the next investigation of
choice?

A. spirometry (lung function tests)
B. arterial blood gas
C. pulse oximetry
D. chest CT scan
E. PEFR

262. What is the best treatment for his condition?

A. prednisolone
B. salbutamol inhaler
C. beclometasone inhaler
D. ipratropium inhaler
E. antituberculous chemotherapy

263. A 60-year-old man is found to have a BP of 170/100. He also
has a history of asthma. What is the most appropriate drug
of choice?

A. furosemide (frusemide)
B. atenolol
C. GTN spray
D. enalapril
E. hydralazine

264. The following medication may be offered to a man suffering from alcoholism EXCEPT:

A. vitamin B complex
B. thiamine
C. diazepam
D. heminevrin
E. acamprosate

265. The following blood tests should routinely be offered to IV drug abusers EXCEPT:

A. HIV
B. hepatitis C
C. hepatitis B
D. LFTs
E. hepatitis A

266. A 40-year-old man presents complaining of an episode of blacking out behind the wheel of his car. The following advice should be given to the patient EXCEPT:

A. not to drive
B. to leave the door unlocked when bathing
C. not to take hot baths
D. not to iron
E. never to be alone

267. The following blood tests should be arranged for this patient EXCEPT:

A. FBC
B. serum calcium
C. serum glucose
D. cardiac isoenzymes
E. ESR

268. A 55-year-old woman presents with severe heartburn. The pain is retrosternal and worse on stooping and after large meals. Initial investigations should include all of the following EXCEPT:

A. FBC
B. ESR
C. *Helicobacter pylori* antibody test
D. folate and B_{12} levels
E. endoscopy

269. Initial management may include each of the following EXCEPT:

A. quit smoking
B. use antacids
C. start esomeprazole
D. start lansoprazole
E. start triple therapy

270. You are on your way to hospital to do a night shift and find an unconscious man on the street. He is unkempt and has needle tracks on his arms and neck. He has pinpoint pupils. He is not arousable. There is no one else on the street. The most appropriate action would be:

A. confirm the patient is breathing, place him in the recovery position and call 999
B. give 2 breaths and call 999 on your mobile to alert the paramedics that it is a likely drug overdose
C. check the patient is breathing and has a pulse and proceed to work
D. run into the hospital and grab a stretcher
E. undress the man to examine him properly for signs of trauma

271. He is transported to your Casualty department. The next step is:

A. administer naloxone IM only after confirmation of presence of opiates in urine
B. administer naloxone IM immediately
C. administer glucagon IM
D. administer IV fluids
E. arrange for urgent CT scan of the head

272. Risk screen for danger to others includes the presence of the following EXCEPT:

A. morbid jealousy
B. hallucinations giving instructions
C. thought disorder
D. lack of remorse about past history of violence
E. violent fantasies

273. A 50-year-old man requests hepatitis B vaccination. Pre Hep B vaccine blood results are:

– Hep B surface antigen
– Hep B core IgM
– Hep Be antigen
+ Hep Be antibody
+ Hep B core antibody (total)
+ Hep B surface antibody

How do you interpret this result?

A. The patient has natural immunity to hepatitis B and does not require vaccination.
B. The patient has had infection with hepatitis B some time in the past.
C. The patient has an acute infection with hepatitis B.
D. The patient is a chronic carrier of high infectivity.
E. The patient is a chronic carrier of low infectivity.

274. The drug of choice for scabies is:

A. permethrin cream
B. malathion lotion
C. crotamiton
D. ketoconazole
E. mebendazole

275. Scabies is transmitted through:

A. bedding
B. towels
C. direct skin contact
D. clothing
E. hair

276. Causes of transient loss of consciousness include all of the following EXCEPT:

A. reflex-mediated syncope
B. aortic stenosis
C. second degree heart block
D. subarachnoid haemorrhage
E. hyperglycaemia

277. A 40-year-old man complains of constant, right-sided headache with severe throbbing orbital pain. The pain lasts for an hour. He also complains of watery eyes and runny nose. He has had several episodes in the last few months and is worried he may have a brain tumour. The most likely diagnosis is:

A. acute sinusitis
B. migraine headache
C. cluster headache
D. orbital cellulitis
E. hayfever

278. A 65-year-old woman complains of severe right-sided headache, centred in the eye, with nausea and vomiting. On examination the conjunctiva is injected with a cloudy anterior chamber. The globe is firm and tender. The most likely diagnosis is:

A. acute sinusitis
B. temporal arteritis
C. acute narrow angle glaucoma
D. trigeminal neuralgia
E. periorbital abscess

279. A 50-year-old man complains of squeezing substernal chest pain when walking the dog in the morning. The attack peaks at 10 minutes and stops at rest. The most likely diagnosis is:

A. oesophageal spasm
B. costochondritis
C. acute myocardial infarction
D. stable angina
E. reflux oesophagitis

280. The risk factors for coronary artery disease include all of the following EXCEPT:

A. tobacco
B. alcohol
C. raised LDL cholesterol
D. diabetes
E. hypertension

281. A 30-year-old man presents with substernal chest pain and shortness of breath. On examination he has a loud sytolic ejection murmur. Valsalva manoeuvre increases the murmur and leg raising decreases the murmur and symptoms. The most likely diagnosis is:

A. mitral valve prolapse
B. hypertrophic cardiomyopathy
C. pericarditis
D. aortic dissection
E. stable angina

282. A 22-year-old man presents with severe, sharp chest pain that worsens with breathing. He has shallow breathing and leans towards the left side. Temperature is 39°C, BP is 100/60 and pulse is 120. White cell count is raised with neutrophilia. Chest x-ray is normal. The most likely diagnosis is:

A. pulmonary embolus
B. pleurodynia
C. tension pneumothorax
D. pericarditis
E. costochondritis

283. Initial management for coma in the emergency setting includes all of the following EXCEPT:

A. 50% dextrose, 50 ml IV
B. 2 mg naloxone IV
C. 100 mg thiamine IV
D. assess airway, breathing and circulation
E. skull x-ray

284. The patient is still unresponsive. The left pupil is now dilated and unresponsive. The next step is:

A. obtain an urgent neurosurgical consult and consider mannitol
B. administer IV broad-spectrum antibiotics
C. perform a lumbar puncture
D. arrange an urgent EEG
E. arrange an urgent MRI scan of the head

285. A 40-year-old woman presents comatose. On examination she has a left mastectomy scar. ECG shows a shortened QT interval. The diagnosis is:

A. hypernatraemia
B. hypercalcaemia
C. Addison's disease
D. hypoglycaemia
E. hypermagnesaemia

286. A 30-year-old woman presents with severe lethargy, weakness and abdominal pain. On examination there is hyperpigmentation of the skin folds and breast areolar areas. Blood tests reveal hypoglycaemia and hyperkalaemia. The most likely diagnosis is:

A. conversion disorder
B. Cushing's disease
C. Addison's disease
D. myxoedema
E. uraemia

287. Beck's triad is:

A. hypotension, muffled heart sounds and jugular vein distension
B. jugular vein distension, hypertension and peripheral oedema
C. pericardial rub, hypotension and jugular vein distension
D. increasing blood pressure, decreasing pulse rate and shallow breathing
E. jaundice, rigors and tender hepatomegaly

288. Lyme disease is associated with:

A. *Borrelia burgdorferi*
B. *Rickettsia rickettsii*
C. *Coxiella burneti*
D. *Leptospira interrogans*
E. *Borrelia recurrentis*

289. Treatment for Lyme disease is:

A. tetracycline
B. penicillin
C. erythromycin
D. imipenem
E. ciprofloxacin

290. The following conditions may be treated with chemotherapy EXCEPT:

A. choriocarcinoma
B. Hodgkin's disease
C. testicular carcinoma
D. Wilm's tumour
E. adenocarcinoma of the stomach

291. Bone metastasis may occur with the following carcinomas EXCEPT:

A. breast
B. prostate
C. thyroid
D. adrenal
E. renal

292. Treatment options for prostate carcinoma include all of the following EXCEPT:

A. local radiotherapy
B. TURP
C. chemotherapy
D. cyproterone acetate
E. orchidectomy

293. Crohn's disease is associated with all of the following EXCEPT:

A. rose-thorn ulcers on barium enema
B. cobblestoning on barium enema
C. perianal abscess
D. loss of haustra on barium enema
E. lymphoma

294. The most common cause of a breast mass in women under 30 is:

A. fibrocystic disease
B. fibroadenoma
C. cystosarcoma phylloides
D. breast abscess
E. lipoma

295. Management of deep venous thrombosis include all of the following EXCEPT:

    A. check platelet count every 3 days
    B. aim for PTT at least 1.5 times normal
    C. elevate lower extremity
    D. give loading dose of 5000 units of heparin followed by heparin infusion of up to 2000 units/h
    E. 5000 units SC fragmin bd

296. The most common anterior mediastinal tumour in adults is:

    A. thymoma
    B. lymphoma
    C. mesothelioma
    D. myoma
    E. fibroma

297. A 55-year-old smoker complains of left leg pain when walking. The pain is relieved on rest. You are unable to palpate the DP or PT pulses on the left. The next step is:

    A. measure ankle brachial pressures to determine ABPI
    B. arrange Doppler scan of leg
    C. arrange angiogram
    D. arrange plethysmography
    E. prescribe pentoxifylline

298. Indications for use of octreotide (somatostain analogue) include all of the following EXCEPT:

    A. acromegaly
    B. variceal bleeding
    C. prevention of complications following pancreatic surgery
    D. cystic fibrosis
    E. carcinoid tumour

299. The investigation of choice for diagnosis of acute pancreatitis is:

    A. dynamic CT scan
    B. serum amylase
    C. abdominal ultrasound
    D. urinary amylase
    E. ERCP

300. A 25-year-old woman IV drug abuser presents with overdose on rocks (cocaine). ECG shows supraventricular tachycardia. First-line treatment for SVT is:

A. adenosine
B. amiodarone
C. lidocaine (lignocaine)
D. procainamide
E. verapamil

Medicine EMQs
Theme: Diagnosis of skin lesions

Options

    A Seborrhoeic keratosis
    B Malignant melanoma
    C Café au lait patch
    D Haemangioma
    E Campbell de Morgan spot
    F Keratoacanthoma
    G Solar keratosis
    H Basal cell carcinoma
    I Squamous cell carcinoma
    J Bowen's disease
    K Marjolin's ulcer

For each presentation below, choose the SINGLE most likely diagnosis from the above list of options. Each option may be used once, more than once, or not at all.

1. A 60-year-old man presents with a persistent itchy ulcer on his right cheek. He has had this ulcer for years. The edges are rolled with a central scab that falls off and reforms. The local lymph nodes are not enlarged.

2. A 65-year-old farmer presents with a grey thickened patch of skin on the rim of his left ear. The 1-cm lesion is painless, raised, firm and has not changed in size over many years.

3. A 40-year-old woman presents with a rapidly growing 1-cm lump in the skin of her wrist. The lump is the same colour as her skin but the centre is necrotic. It is freely mobile and rubbery in consistency with a hard core.

4. A newborn baby presents with several 2-cm pale brown macules on the back.

5. A 20-year-old man presents with a chronic paronychia. On examination there is an expanding brown pigmentation present beneath the toenail with enlargement of local lymph nodes.

Theme: Causes of dysphagia

Options

    A Achalasia
    B Pharyngeal pouch
    C Diffuse oesophageal spasm
    D Globus pharyngeus
    E Plummer–Vinson syndrome
    F Carcinoma of the oesophagus
    G Peptic stricture
    H Myasthenia gravis
    I   Swallowed foreign body
    J   Caustic stricture
    K Retrosternal goitre

For each presentation below, choose the SINGLE most likely cause from the above list of options. Each option may be used once, more than once, or not at all.

6. A 32-year-old female presents with progressive dysphagia with regurgitation of fluids. She denies weight loss.

7. A 27-year-old man with a history of depression presents with acute dysphagia. He has a prior history of repeated suicide attempts. There are associated burns in his oropharynx.

8. A 60-year-old woman presents with progressive dysphagia. On examination she has a smooth tongue, koilonychia and suffers from iron-deficiency anaemia.

9. A 65-year-old man presents with regurgitation of food, dysphagia, halitosis and a sensation of a 'lump in the throat'.

10. A 70-year-old man presents with a short history of dysphagia, weight loss and has palpable neck nodes on examination.

Theme: Investigation of weight loss

Options

    A Stool for cysts, ova and parasites
    B Urea and electrolytes
    C Chest x-ray
    D Full blood count
    E Serum glucose
    F Urinalysis
    G Thyroid function tests
    H Ultrasound of abdomen
    I Barium swallow
    J Blood cultures
    K Plasma ACTH and cortisol

For each presentation below, choose the SINGLE most discriminating investigation from the above list of options. Each option may be used once, more than once, or not at all.

11. A 60-year-old man recently treated for renal tuberculosis presents with weight loss, diarrhoea, anorexia, hypotension and is noted to have hyperpigmented buccal mucosa and hand creases.

12. A 50-year-old woman presents with weight loss, increased appetite, sweating, palpitations, preference for cold weather, hot, moist palms and tremors.

13. A 25-year-old man presents with steatorrhoea, diarrhoea and weight loss after eating contaminated food.

14. A 65-year-old man presents with a sudden onset of diabetes, anorexia, weight loss, epigastric and back pain.

15. A 70-year-old woman presents with progressive dysphagia, weight loss and a sensation of food sticking in her throat.

Theme: Investigation of pyrexia of unknown origin

Options

    A Haemoglobin
    B Full blood count
    C Erythrocyte sedimentation rate
    D Lymph node biopsy
    E CT scan of the chest
    F Stool cultures
    G Mantoux test
    H Monospot
    I   Echocardiography for vegetations
    J Kveim test
    K HIV antibody titres

For each presentation below, choose the SINGLE most discriminating investigation from the above list of options. Each option may be used once, more than once, or not at all.

16. A 17-year-old boy presents with a 2-week history of fever, malaise and cervical lymphadenopathy. On examination there is tenderness in the right upper quadrant of the abdomen and the sclerae are yellow.

17. A 25-year-old male drug addict presents with a low-grade fever, malaise, a change in heart murmur, splinter haemorrhages in the nail beds and Osler's nodes in the finger pulp.

18. A 54-year-old man presents with a 2-month history of unilateral enlargement of his right tonsil, fluctuating pyrexia and multiple neck nodes.

19. A 25-year-old woman presents with fever, malaise, erythema nodosum and polyarthralgia. Chest x-ray reveals mediastinal hilar lymphadenopathy.

20. A 29-year-old IV drug abuser presents with fever and a neck node discharging a cheesy, malodorous substance.

Theme: Treatment of meningitis

Options

    A Benzylpenicillin
    B Chloramphenicol
    C Ampicillin
    D Rifampicin, ethambutol, isoniazid and pyrazinamide
    E Amphotericin B and flucytosine
    F Gentamicin
    G Erythromycin
    H Cefotaxime
    I Oral rifampicin
    J Vancomycin
    K Supportive

For each case below, choose the SINGLE most appropriate treatment from the above list of options. Each option may be used once, more than once, or not at all.

21. A 3-year-old girl presents with acute onset of pyrexia, nausea and vomiting. Lumbar puncture reveals high protein and polymorph count and low glucose. Gram-negative bacilli are present in the smear and culture.

22. A 40-year-old man presents with fever and meningeal signs. Lumbar puncture reveals $20/mm^3$ mononuclear cells, 2 g/L of protein and a glucose level half the plasma level. There are no organisms in the smear.

23. A 17-year-old girl presents with fever, odd behaviour, purpura and conjunctival petechiae. Lumbar puncture reveals Gram-negative cocci.

24. A 22-year-old man presents with fever, headache and drowsiness. Lumbar puncture reveals 1000 mononuclear cells/mm^3, 0.5 g/L of protein and a glucose greater than two-thirds of the plasma glucose level. Organisms are absent.

25. The 25-year-old husband of a patient admitted with pyogenic meningitis admits to having oral contact with his wife and is anxious.

Theme: Causes of anaemia

Options

    A Vitamin B_{12} deficiency
    B Iron deficiency
    C Sickle-cell anaemia
    D Pernicious anaemia
    E Autoimmune haemolytic anaemia
    F Hypothyroidism
    G Sideroblastic anaemia
    H Anaemia of chronic disease
    I Glucose-6-phosphate dehydrogenase deficiency
    J Thalassaemia
    K Coeliac disease

For each presentation below, choose the SINGLE most likely cause from the above list of options. Each option may be used once, more than once, or not at all.

26. An 8-year-old boy presents with painful swelling of the hands and feet, jaundice and anaemia. He is noted to have splenomegaly. Blood film has target cells.

27. A 6-month-old baby boy presents with severe anaemia and failure to thrive. Blood film shows target cells, hypochromic and microcytic cells. HbF persists.

28. A 40-year-old woman presents with fatigue, dyspnoea, paraesthesiae and a sore, red tongue. Blood film shows hypersegmented polymorphs, an MCV > 110 fl and a low Hb.

29. A 60-year-old man post gastrectomy presents with macrocytic anaemia. He drinks alcohol regularly.

30. A 22-year-old Greek man presents with rapid anaemia and jaundice following treatment of malaria. He is noted to have Heinz bodies.

Theme: Diagnosis of red eye

Options
  A Acute glaucoma
  B Iritis
  C Conjunctivitis
  D Subconjunctival haemorrhage
  E Optic neuritis
  F Conjunctival haemorrhages
  G Scleritis
  H Anterior uveitis
  I Posterior uveitis
  J Retinal haemorrhages

For each patient below, choose the SINGLE most likely diagnosis from the above list of options. Each option may be used once, more than once, or not at all.

31. A 55-year-old woman presents with an entirely red right eye. The iris is injected, and the pupil is fixed and dilated. The intraocular pressure is high.

32. A 20-year-old man presents with a non-tender red eye. On examination the sclera is bright red with a white rim around the limbus. The iris, pupil, cornea and intraocular pressure are normal.

33. A 33-year-old woman presents with a painful red eye. The conjunctival vessels are injected and blanch on pressure. The iris, pupil, cornea and intraocular pressures are normal.

34. A 40-year-old man presents with redness most marked around the cornea. The colour does not blanch on pressure. The iris is injected, and the pupil is small and fixed. The cornea and intraocular pressure are normal.

35. A 20-year-old man with non-specific urethritis and seronegative arthritis is also noted to have red eye associated with Reiter's syndrome.

Theme: Diagnosis of skin manifestations of systemic diseases

Options

    A Erythema nodosum
    B Erythema multiforme
    C Erythema marginatum
    D Erythema chronicum migrans
    E Vitiligo
    F Pyoderma gangrenosum
    G Acquired icthyosis
    H Necrobiosis lipoidica
    I Dermatitis herpetiformis
    J Acanthosis nigricans
    K Pretibial myxoedema

For each patient below, choose the SINGLE most likely skin manifestation from the above list of options. Each option may be used once, more than once, or not at all.

36. A 53-year-old female presents with proptosis, heat intolerance and red oedematous swellings over the lateral malleoli which progress to thickened oedema.

37. A 45-year-old man presents with shiny area on his shins with yellowish skin and telangiectasia. He also suffers from areas of fat necrosis.

38. A 55-year-old female who is advised to eat a gluten-free diet presents with itchy blisters in groups on her knees, elbows and scalp.

39. A 30-year-old man suffering from Crohn's disease presents with a pustule on his leg with a tender red/blue necrotic edge.

40. A 15-year-old female presents with fever and mouth ulcers. She is also noted to have target lesions with a central blister on her palms and soles.

Theme: Diagnosis of eye problems

Options

    A Flame and blot haemorrhages
    B Proliferative retinopathy
    C Xanthelasma
    D Senile cataracts
    E Amaurosis fugax
    F Optic atrophy
    G Periorbital abscess
    H Corneal arcus
    I Kayser–Fleischer rings
    J Hypertensive fundus
    K Lens opacities
    L Background retinopathy

For each patient below, choose the SINGLE most likely diagnosis from the above list of options. Each option may be used once, more than once, or not at all.

41. A 65-year-old male with IDDM is noted to have a white ring in his cornea surrounding his iris.

42. A 55-year-old man complains of 'a curtain passing over his eyes'. Carotid bruits are present on auscultation.

43. A 12-year-old boy, following an episode of sinusitis, complains of persistent pain behind the right eye with eyelid swelling and diminished vision.

44. A 40-year-old woman complains of pruritus, jaundice and finger clubbing. There are bright yellow plaques on both eyelids.

45. A 30-year-old man is noted to have rubeosis iridis, cotton wool spots and cluster haemorrhages.

Theme: Diagnosis of haematological diseases

Options

A Hereditary spherocytosis
B Myeloid metaplasia
C Uraemia
D Iron-deficiency anaemia
E Sickle-cell anaemia
F Megaloblastic anaemia
G Chronic granulocytic leukaemia
H Infectious mononucleosis
I Chronic lymphocytic leukaemia
J Acute myeloid leukaemia
K Multiple myeloma
L Hodgkin's disease

For each blood smear below, choose the SINGLE most likely diagnosis from the above list of options. Each option may be used once, more than once, or not at all.

46. A 25-year-old female presents with an enlarged, painless lymph node in the neck. She also reports fever and weight loss. Peripheral blood smear shows Reed–Sternberg cells with a bilobed, mirror-imaged nucleus.

47. A 70-year-old man presents with bone pain, anaemia and renal failure. Bone marrow reveals an abundance of malignant plasma cells.

48. A 10-year-old boy presents with swelling of the hands and feet and anaemia. Peripheral blood smear reveals target cells and elongated crescent-shaped red blood cells.

49. A 50-year-old man with IDDM presents with a 'lemon' tinge to the skin, itching, peripheral oedema, pleural effusions and anaemia. Peripheral blood smear reveals numerous Burr cells, red blood cells with spiny projections.

50. A 65-year-old woman presents with anaemia. She has koilonychia and atrophic glossitis. Blood smear reveals microcytic, hypochromic blood cells.

Theme: Diagnosis of heart conditions

Options

    A Anterolateral MI
    B Left ventricular failure
    C Atrial fibrillation
    D Acute pulmonary embolism
    E Acute pericarditis
    F Mitral stenosis
    G Right ventricular failure
    H Hypokalaemia
    I Hypocalcaemia
    J Aortic regurgitation
    K Inferolateral MI

For each presentation below, choose the SINGLE most likely diagnosis from the above list of options. Each option may be used once, more than once, or not at all.

51. A 60-year-old man presents with chest pain radiating down the left arm. 12-lead electrocardiogram reveals Q waves in II, III and AVf with T wave changes in V5 and V6.

52. A 50-year-old woman presents with a fast heart rate with an irregular rhythm. There are no P waves on the electrocardiogram. She states that she has lost weight recently and is 'nervous'. She also suffers from palpitations.

53. On auscultation a patient is noted to have a rumbling diastolic murmur at the apex. The murmur is accentuated during exercise.

54. A 60-year-old man on digitalis and diuretics presents with weakness and lethargy. Electrocardiogram shows flat T waves and prominent U waves.

55. A 65-year-old man with chronic bronchitis presents with a raised JVP, hepatomegaly, ankle and sacral oedema.

Theme: Causes of hypertension

Options

A Coarctation of the aorta
B Cushing's syndrome
C Phaeochromocytoma
D Primary hyperaldosteronism
E Polyarteritis nodosa
F Polycystic kidneys
G Acromegaly
H Pre-eclampsia
I Essential hypertension
J Renal artery stenosis
K Chronic glomerulonephritis

For each presentation below, choose the SINGLE most likely cause from the above list of options. Each option may be used once, more than once, or not at all.

56. A 45-year-old woman presents with hypertension and confusion. She has truncal obesity, proximal myopathy and osteoporosis. The 24-hour urinary free cortisol level is raised.

57. A 35-year-old man presents with hypertension and complains of tingling in his fingers. He has an enlarged tongue and prognathism. The glucose tolerance curve is diabetic.

58. A 45-year-old woman with disproportionately long limbs presents with hypertension. Blood pressure is different on both arms and lower in the legs.

59. A 40-year-old man post thyroidectomy for medullary thyroid carcinoma presents with hypertension and complains of attacks of severe headache and palpitations. He is noted to have glycosuria.

60. A 50-year-old man presents with hypertension, haematuria and abdominal pain. A large kidney is palpated on examination, and the diagnosis is confirmed on ultrasound.

Theme: Causes of peripheral neuropathy

Options

    A Carcinomatous neuropathy
    B Side-effect of drug therapy
    C Diabetic neuropathy
    D Vitamin B_{12} deficiency
    E Vitamin B_1 deficiency
    F Polyarteritis nodosa
    G Guillain–Barré syndrome
    H Amyloidosis
    I Sarcoidosis
    J Industrial poisoning
    K Porphyria

For each patient below, choose the SINGLE most likely diagnosis from the above list of options. Each option may be used once, more than once, or not at all.

61. A 50-year-old man presents with distal sensory neuropathy affecting the lower limbs in a 'stocking' distribution and is noted to have Charcot's joints. The ankle reflex is absent.

62. A 55-year-old man who drinks heavily presents with numbness and paraesthesiae in his feet. He complains of 'walking on cotton wool'.

63. A 40-year-old man, who is being treated with chemotherapy for lymphoma, presents with peripheral paraesthesiae, loss of deep tendon reflexes and abdominal bloating.

64. A 45-year-old woman presents with peripheral neuropathy. There is bilateral hilar gland enlargement on chest x-ray. The Mantoux test is negative. She also suffers from polyarthralgia and has tender red, raised lesions on her shin.

65. A 25-year-old man presents with paraesthesiae followed by a flaccid paralysis of his limbs and face. He has a history of a recent upper respiratory tract infection.

Theme: Diagnosis of pulmonary diseases

Options

A Pneumoconiosis
B Cystic fibrosis
C Mycoplasma pneumonia
D Adult respiratory distress syndrome
E Pulmonary contusion
F Carcinoma of the bronchus
G Pancoast's tumour
H Bilateral bronchopneumonia
I Sarcoidosis
J Tuberculosis

For each case below, choose the SINGLE most likely diagnosis from the above list of options. Each option may be used once, more than once, or not at all.

66. A 30-year-old woman presents with fever, pharyngitis, and cough. Chest x-ray shows widespread bilateral patchy consolidation. Cold agglutinins are detected.

67. A 40-year-old alcoholic presents with repeated small haemoptysis and cough with mucoid sputum. Chest x-ray shows right upper lobe consolidation and a large central cavity. The Heaf test is positive.

68. A 60-year-old man presents with dyspnoea and cough. X-ray shows extensive pulmonary fibrosis, bilateral pleural thickening and pleural calcification.

69. A 14-year-old boy presents with repeated lower tract respiratory infections. On examination there is finger clubbing. He suffers from weight loss and steatorrhoea. The x-ray shows bronchial wall thickening, ring shadows of bronchiectasis and widespread ill-defined shadowing.

70. A 40-year-old man presents with cough and haemoptysis. The x-ray shows a right hilar mass and a patch of consolidation in the right upper lobe laterally.

Theme: Treatment of hypertension

Options

    A Atenolol
    B Bendrofluazide
    C Furosemide (frusemide)
    D Methyldopa
    E Amlodipine
    F Nifedipine
    G Hydralazine
    H Captopril
    I Sodium nitroprusside
    J Lisinopril
    K Non-drug treatment

For each patient below, choose the SINGLE most appropriate treatment from the above list of options. Each option may be used once, more than once, or not at all.

71. A 60-year-old man presents with a BP of 165/95. He is asymptomatic, and all investigations are normal.

72. A 55-year-old insulin dependent diabetic presents to his GP with a BP of 170/110. The blood pressure is consistently high on subsequent visits despite conservative measures. Blood tests are normal.

73. A 50-year-old man with asthma presents to his GP with a BP of 180/120. All underlying causes have been excluded.

74. A 60-year-old man is brought into Accident and Emergency complaining of severe headaches. On arrival he has a seizure. BP is noted to be 220/140 and on fundoscopic examination, there is papilloedema.

75. A 66-year-old man on atenolol 100 mg od continues to have a diastolic blood pressure of 115. He also takes allopurinol. A second drug is recommended.

Theme: Causes of splenomegaly

Options

      A   Typhoid
      B   Gaucher's disease
      C   Malaria
      D   Schistosomiasis
      E   Lymphoma
      F   Leishmaniasis
      G   Idiopathic thrombocytopenic purpura
      H   Polycythaemia rubra vera
      I   Felty's syndrome
      J   Leptospirosis
      K   Chronic myeloid leukaemia

For each case below, choose the SINGLE most likely cause from the above list of options. Each option may be used once, more than once, or not at all.

76. A 20-year-old man presents acutely with fever, jaundice, purpura, injected conjunctiva and painful calves after swimming outdoors.

77. A 26-year-old man recently returned from a trip to India presents with intermittent fevers, cough, diarrhoea, epistaxis and massive splenomegaly.

78. A 22-year-old female presents with epistaxis and easy bruising. On examination the spleen is palpable.

79. A 30-year-old Jewish man presents with incidental splenomegaly on a routine physical examination at his GP's clinic. Serum acid phosphatase is elevated. He admits to having episodes of bone pain. His uncle also has an enlarged spleen.

80. A 60-year-old female with rheumatoid arthritis presents with splenomegaly. Full blood count shows a white count of 1500/mm^3.

Theme: Causes of haematuria

Options

    A Ureteric calculus
    B Acute pyelonephritis
    C Benign prostatic hypertrophy
    D Acute cystitis
    E Malaria
    F Carcinoma of the kidney
    G Bladder carcinoma
    H Bilharzia
    I Prostate carcinoma
    J Renal vein thrombosis
    K Acute intermittent porphyria

For each of the cases below, choose the SINGLE most likely cause from the above list of options. Each option may be used once, more than once, or not at all.

81. An 18-year-old female started on oral contraceptives complains of colicky abdominal pain and vomiting and fever. Urine is positive for red blood cells and protein. She develops progressive weakness in her extremities.

82. A 60-year-old man presents with intermittent colicky loin pain and night sweats. He has profuse haematuria with passage of blood clots. He is noted to have a varicocoele and peripheral oedema. He admits to loss of energy and weight loss.

83. A 25-year-old woman presents with fever and tachycardia. On examination the renal angle is very tender. Urine is cloudy and blood-stained.

84. A 40-year-old man complains of severe colicky loin pain that radiates to his scrotum. He is noted to have microscopic haematuria. No masses are palpated.

85. A 60-year-old man complains of increased frequency of micturition with suprapubic ache. Urine is cloudy and mahogany brown in colour.

Theme: Causes of abnormal electrocardiograms

Options

A Hypokalaemia
B Hyperkalaemia
C Hypocalcaemia
D Hypercalcaemia
E Myocardial ischaemia
F Inferior MI
G Acute pulmonary embolism
H Acute pericarditis
I Atrial fibrillation
J Myxoedema
K Digitalis intoxication
L Inferolateral MI

For each case below, choose the SINGLE most likely cause of ECG changes from the above list of options. Each option may be used once, more than once, or not at all.

86. A 60-year-old woman taking furosemide (frusemide) is noted to have 'U' waves in leads V3 and V4.

87. A 50-year-old man presents with fever and chest pain. He has a history of angina. ECG reveals concave elevation of the ST segments in leads II, V5 and V6.

88. A 55-year-old man presents with chest pain and dyspnoea. ECG reveals 'Q' waves in leads III and AVf and inverted 'T' waves in leads V1–3.

89. A 55-year-old woman who has undergone thyroidectomy is noted to have an ECG with a QT interval of 0.50.

90. A 60-year-old woman presents with hoarseness. She is a smoker and is on prozac. Pulse rate is 44/min and ECG is noted for sinus bradycardia and reduced amplitude of P, QRS and T waves in all leads.

Theme: Treatment of medical emergencies

Options

    A Cardioversion
    B Cricothyroidotomy
    C Needle thoracocentesis
    D Needle pericardiocentesis
    E Insertion of chest drain
    F Endotracheal intubation
    G Defibrillation
    H Needle aspiration
    I Intravenous heparin
    J Intramuscular epinephrine (adrenaline)
    K Intravenous aminophylline

For each case below, choose the SINGLE most appropriate treatment from the above list of options. Each option may be used once, more than once, or not at all.

91. A 45-year-old woman presents with acute dyspnoea and stridor. The tongue is swollen.

92. A 20-year-old student presents with respiratory distress and pleuritic pain. On examination there are distended neck veins and no breath sounds over the right lung field.

93. A 30-year-old man presents with chest pain. There are distended neck veins and muffled heart sounds. Blood pressure is 80/50.

94. A 55-year-old woman presents with stridor and difficulty swallowing following thyroidectomy. On examination there is a tense swelling over the surgical site.

95. A 30-year-old female presents with acute dyspnoea and pleuritic pain. Regular medications include salbutamol inhaler and Microgynon. Respiratory rate is 30 with a small volume rapid pulse rate of 110 and a BP of 80/50. The JVP is raised Chest x-ray is normal. Electrocardiogram shows sinus tachycardia.

Theme: Investigation of liver disease

Options

    A Mitochondrial antibodies
    B Serum iron and total iron-binding capacity
    C Serum copper and caeruloplasmin
    D Serum bilirubin and liver function tests
    E HBs antigen
    F Hepatitis C IgG
    G Antibodies against nuclei and actin
    H Antibodies to HAV
    I   Gamma-glutamyl transferase level
    J Alpha-1-antitrypsin

For each presentation below, choose the SINGLE most discriminating investigation from the above list of options. Each option may be used once, more than once, or not at all.

96. A 60-year-old man with emphysema presents with liver disease. The sputum is purulent and found to contain elastases and proteases.

97. A 50-year-old woman presents with pruritus and jaundice. She complains of dry eyes and mouth. Xanthelasma and hepatosplenomegaly are present on examination.

98. A 50-year-old well-bronzed man presents with a loss of libido. On examination hepatomegaly is noted. He takes Humulin and Actrapid insulin.

99. A 22-year-old man presents with tremor and dysarthria. On examination he is noted to have a greenish-brown pigment at the corneoscleral junction.

100. A 30-year-old woman presents with acute hepatitis. She is pyrexial, jaundiced, with hepatosplenomegaly, bruising and migratory polyarthritis. She is noted to have a goitre.

Theme: Causes of back pain

Options

    A Multiple myeloma
    B Secondary prostate disease
    C Osteomyelitis
    D Ankylosing spondylitis
    E Sarcoidosis
    F Lupus
    G Reiter's disease
    H Lumbar prolapse and sciatica
    I Spondylolisthesis
    J Spinal stenosis
    K Paget's disease
    L Osteoarthritis

For each presentation below, choose the SINGLE most likely cause from the above list of options. Each option may be used once, more than once, or not at all.

101. A 30-year-old female complains of sudden and severe back pain. Her back has 'gone'. She walks with a compensated scoliosis. On examination she has pain from the buttock to her ankle and sensory loss over the sole of her left foot and calf.

102. A 50-year-old man presents with back pain radiating down the back of both his legs. The pain is aggravated by walking and relieved by resting or leaning forward. On examination he has limited straight-leg raise and absent ankle reflexes.

103. A 50-year-old woman presents with backache. She is noted to have a normocytic, normochromic anaemia and a high ESR.

104. A 60-year-old man presents with lumbar spine bone pain and pain in his hips. The serum alkaline phosphatase is 1000 IU/L. The calcium and phosphate levels are normal. He is hard of hearing.

105. A 20-year-old man complains of lower back pain radiating down the back of both his legs. On x-ray the vertebrae are square and tramline. ESR is elevated.

Theme: Investigation of urinary tract obstruction

Options

    A Excretion urography
    B Ultrasonography
    C Dynamic scintigraphy
    D Cystourethroscopy
    E Plain KUB film
    F Pressure-flow studies
    G Retrograde ureterography
    H Urethrography
    I Serum urea and electrolytes
    J Urinalysis
    K Midstream specimen for culture

For each presentation below, choose the SINGLE most discriminating investigation from the above list of options. Each option may be used once more than once, or not at all.

106. A 65-year-old man with diabetes presents with a painless distended bladder. On digital rectal examination, his prostate is not enlarged.

107. A 40-year-old man presents with severe colicky loin pain radiating to his testicle. Plain abdominal x-ray is unremarkable. He has microscopic haematuria.

108. A 50-year-old man presents with severe oliguria post kidney transplant.

109. A 60-year-old man post thyroidectomy presents with painful urinary retention. There is some difficulty in catheterisation with a 900-ml residual. Digital rectal examination reveals a smooth, enlarged prostate.

110. A 60-year-old man presents with malaise, back pain, normochromic anaemia, uraemia, and a high ESR. He has known carcinoma of the colon.

Theme: Diagnosis of chronic joint pain

Options

    A Gout
    B Septic arthritis
    C Rheumatoid arthritis
    D Osteoarthritis
    E Pyrophosphate arthropathy
    F Systemic lupus erythematosus
    G Systemic sclerosis
    H Polymyositis
    I Still's disease
    J Multiple myeloma
    K Sjögren's syndrome

For each case below, choose the SINGLE most likely diagnosis from the above list of options. Each option may be used once, more than once, or not at all.

111. A 70-year-old woman complains of arthritis in the fingers and big toe. On examination there are bony swellings of the first carpometacarpal joints. The proximal interphalangeal joints and metatarsophalangeal joint are also affected.

112. A 45-year-old woman presents with swellings and stiffness of her fingers. On examination she has sausage-like fingers with flexion deformities. She is noted to have a beaked nose. She takes Losec. X-ray of her hands reveals deposits of calcium around the fingers and erosion of the tufts of the distal phalanges.

113. A 40-year-old woman complains of arthritic hands, weakness in her arms and difficulty swallowing. She has trouble carrying her shopping. On examination the small joints of her hands are swollen. Blood tests reveal a raised ESR and a normocytic anaemia. Serum antinuclear antibodies and rheumatoid factor tests are positive.

114. A 50-year-old woman on thyroxine for hypothyroidism presents with stiff swollen knees. Aspiration of the synovial fluid reveals positively birefringent crystals.

115. An elderly man presents with a red, warm, swollen metatarsal phalangeal joint following a right total hip replacement operation.

Theme: Causes of finger clubbing

Options

    A Bronchial carcinoma
    B Bronchiectasis
    C Lung abscess
    D Empyema
    E Cryptogenic fibrosing alveolitis
    F Mesothelioma
    G Cyanotic heart disease
    H Subacute bacterial endocarditis
    I Cirrhosis
    J Inflammatory bowel disease
    K Coeliac disease
    L GI lymphoma

For each presentation below, choose the SINGLE most likely associative cause from the above list of options. Each option may be used once, more than once, or not at all.

116. A 35-year-old heroin addict presents with fever, night sweats and haematuria. On examination he is noted to have a heart murmur and finger clubbing.

117. A 50-year-old farmer is noted to have a dry cough, exertional dyspnoea, weight loss, arthralgia and finger clubbing. On x-ray there is bilateral diffuse reticulonodular shadowing at the bases.

118. A 60-year-old man presents with severe chest pain, dyspnoea and finger clubbing. He admits to asbestos exposure 20 years ago. He denies smoking. Chest x-ray reveals a unilateral pleural effusion.

119. A 30-year-old woman presents with fever, diarrhoea and crampy abdominal pain. She is noted to have finger clubbing, anal fissures and a skin tag.

120. A 50-year-old man presents with haematemesis. He is noted to have finger clubbing, gynaecomastia and spider naevi.

Theme: Causes of headache

Options

A Meningitis
B Migraine headache
C Cluster headache
D Tension headache
E Subarachnoid haemorrhage
F Sinusitis
G Benign intracranial hypertension
H Cervical spondylosis
I Giant-cell arteritis
J Otitis media
K Transient ischaemic attack

For each case below, choose the SINGLE most likely cause from the above list of options. Each option may be used once, more than once, or not at all.

121. A 25-year-old female presents with episodes of unilateral throbbing headache, nausea and vomiting. She states that it is aggravated by light. The episodes seem to occur prior to her menstruation.

122. A 40-year-old man presents with severe pain around his right eye with eyelid swelling lasting 20 minutes. He has had several attacks during the past weeks. The attacks are worse at night.

123. A 10-year-old boy presents with fever, headache, left eye pain and swelling. He described his vision as blurry. He has recently recovered from a cold.

124. A 60-year-old female presents with bitemporal headache, unilateral blurry vision and pain on combing her hair. The ESR is elevated.

125. A 30-year-old obese female presents with headache and diplopia. On examination she has papilloedema. She is alert with no focal symptoms and signs.

Theme: Diagnosis of cardiovascular disease

Options

A Aortic regurgitation
B Mitral stenosis
C Mitral regurgitation
D Aortic stenosis
E Atrial myxoma
F Tricuspid regurgitation
G Pulmonary stenosis
H Atrial septal defect
I Ventricular septal defect
J Fallot's tetralogy
K Patent ductus arteriosus
L Coarctation of the aorta
M Eisenmenger's syndrome

For each patient below, choose the SINGLE most likely diagnosis from the above list of options. Each option may be used once, more than once, or not at all.

126. A 35-year-old pregnant woman presents to her GP for her first prenatal check-up. He notes that her blood pressure differs in both arms and is lower in the legs.

127. A 13-year-old boy presents with dyspnoea and short stature. He is noted to have finger clubbing. The chest x-ray reveals a boot-shaped heart and a large aorta.

128. A preterm baby presents with tachypnoea and expiratory grunting. The baby is noted to have a continuous machinery-like murmur in the second left intercostal space and posteriorly. The ECG is normal.

129. A 33-year-old woman with Marfan's syndrome is noted to have a fixed wide split of the second heart sound. The ECG shows a partial right bundle branch block with right axis deviation and right ventricular hypertrophy.

130. A 40-year-old drug addict is noted to have a pansystolic murmur at the bottom of the sternum. Giant 'cv' waves are present in the jugular venous pulse.

Theme: Causes of pneumonia

Options

A Chlamydia psittaci
B Streptococcus pneumoniae
C Mycoplasma pneumoniae
D Haemophilus influenzae
E Staphylococcus aureus
F Legionella pneumophila
G Coxiella burneti
H Pseudomonas aeruginosa
I Pneumocystis carinii
J Aspergillus fumigatus
K Cytomegalovirus
L Actinomyces israelii
M Klebsiella pneumoniae

For each case below, choose the SINGLE most likely cause from the above list of options. Each option may be used once, more than once, or not at all.

131. A pet-shop owner presents with high, swinging fever, cough and malaise. He has scanty rose spots over his abdomen. The chest x-ray reveals diffuse pneumonia.

132. A 70-year-old alcoholic man presents with sudden onset of purulent productive cough. The chest x-ray shows consolidation of the left upper lobe.

133. A 10-year-old boy with cystic fibrosis presents with pneumonia.

134. A 30-year-old man with AIDS presents with fever, dry cough and dyspnoea. The x-ray shows diffuse bilateral alveolar and interstitial shadowing beginning in the perihilar regions and spreading outward.

135. A 20-year-old male IV drug abuser presents with breathlessness and cough. The x-ray reveals patchy areas of consolidation with abscess formation.

Theme: Causes of visual disturbance

Options

    A *Chlamydia trachomatis*
    B Side-effect of medication
    C Giant-cell arteritis
    D Diabetic retinopathy
    E Multiple sclerosis
    F Vitamin B_{12} deficiency
    G Horner's syndrome
    H Neurosyphilis
    I Myasthenia gravis
    J Pituitary neoplasm
    K Oculomotor nerve lesion
    L Abducens nerve lesion

For each case below, choose the SINGLE most likely cause from the above list of options. Each option may be used once, more than once, or not at all.

136. A 40-year-old woman presents with blurry vision. On examination, when asked to look to her left, the left eye develops nystagmus, and the right eye fails to adduct. When asked to look to her right, the left eye fails to adduct.

137. A 30-year-old woman is noted to have a small, irregular pupil that is fixed to light but constricts on convergence. Fasting blood glucose is 5 mmol/L.

138. A 24-year-old man presents with unilateral pupillary constriction with slight ptosis and enophthalmos. He is noted to have a cervical rib on x-ray.

139. A 25-year-old man who has sustained head injury in an RTA presents with diplopia on lateral gaze. On examination he has a convergent squint with diplopia when looking to the left side.

140. A 40-year-old man with diabetes presents with a unilateral complete ptosis. The eye is noted to be facing down and out. The pupil is spared.

Theme: Investigation of dementia

Options

    A Chest x-ray
    B Serum calcium level
    C TSH levels and serum T4
    D Full blood count and film
    E Electroencephalogram
    F Lumbar puncture
    G Serum urea
    H Liver function tests
    I   CT scan
    J Serum glucose
    K VDRL
    L HIV serology
    M Serum copper and caeruloplasmin
    N Dietary history
    O Drug levels

For each case below, choose the SINGLE most discriminating investigation from the above list of options. Each option may be used once, more than once, or not at all.

141. A 50-year-old woman who underwent thyroidectomy a week prior now presents with dementia. She also complains of perioral tingling.

142. A 70-year-old man presents with progressive dementia and tremor. On examination he has extensor plantar reflexes and Argyll Robertson pupils.

143. A 40-year-old man with a history of epilepsy presents with progressive dementia with fluctuating levels of consciousness. On examination he has unequal pupils.

144. A 30-year-old homosexual man presents with weight loss, chronic diarrhoea and progressive dementia. On examination he has purple papules on his legs.

145. A 30-year-old man presents with sweating, agitation, tremors and dementia. He admits to binge drinking.

Theme: Causes of vertigo

Options

    A Migraine
    B Vestibular neuronitis
    C Multiple sclerosis
    D Lateral medullary syndrome
    E Wernicke's encephalopathy
    F Vertebrobasilar ischaemia
    G Epilepsy
    H Hypoglycaemia
    I Arrhythmias
    J Menière's disease
    K Acoustic neuroma
    L Postural hypotension

For each case below, choose the SINGLE most likely cause from the above list of options. Each option may be used once, more than once, or not at all.

146. A 40-year-old man presents with vertigo, nausea, and weakness. He also complains of a tingling sensation down his right arm and double vision in one eye. On examination he has loss of central vision, nystagmus and ataxia.

147. A 50-year-old man presents with severe vertigo with vomiting and left-sided facial pain. On examination he has nystagmus on looking to the left. His soft palate is paralysed on the left side and he has analgaesia to pinprick on the left side of the face and right limbs. He also has a left-sided Horner's syndrome.

148. A 50-year-old woman presents with vertigo and unilateral deafness. The attacks of vertigo last for hours and are accompanied by vomiting. On examination she has nystagmus and a low frequency sensorineural hearing loss.

149. A 20-year-old man presents with sudden onset of vertigo and vomiting. He denies tinnitus or hearing loss. He had an upper respiratory tract infection a week prior.

150. A 60-year-old man presents with vertigo brought on by turning his head, ataxia, dysarthria and nystagmus.

Theme: Treatment of respiratory diseases

Options

    A Beta$_2$-adrenoreceptor agonist
    B Intravenous aminophylline
    C Erythromycin
    D Tobramycin and carbenicillin
    E Ciprofloxacin
    F Co-trimoxazole
    G Rifampicin and isoniazid
    H Prednisolone
    I Cyclophosphamide
    J Plasmapharesis
    K Tetracycline

For each presentation below, choose the SINGLE most appropriate treatment from the above list of options. Each option may be used once, more than once, or not at all.

151. A 12-year-old boy with cystic fibrosis presents with a chest infection. The boy also suffers from mild renal failure.

152. A 40-year-old mental inpatient presents with dry cough and confusion. Blood tests reveal lymphopenia and hyponatraemia. Chest x-ray shows right-sided lobar shadowing.

153. A 10-year-old boy presents with wheezing attacks and episodic shortness of breath. Peak expiratory flow rate is 400 L/min.

154. A 40-year-old male presents with rhinorrhoea, cough, haemoptysis and pleuritic pain. Chest x-ray shows multiple nodules.

155. A 60-year-old farmer presents with fever, cough and shortness of breath. He had been forking hay that morning. Chest x-ray shows fluffy nodular shadows in the upper zones.

Theme: Investigation of haemoptysis

Options

      A Full blood count
      B Clotting studies
      C Bronchography
      D Chest x-ray
      E 12-lead electrocardiogram
      F Anti-nuclear antibodies and free DNA
      G Anti-glomerular basement antibody in the serum
      H CT scan of the chest
      I Heaf test
      J Urinalysis
      K Pulmonary angiogram
      L Tissue biopsy
      M Sputum cytology

For each case below, choose the SINGLE most discriminating investigation from the above list of options. Each option may be used once, more than once, or not at all.

156. A 40-year-old man presents with recurrent epistaxis, haemoptysis and haematuria. On examination he has a nasal septal perforation and nodules on chest x-ray.

157. A 30-year-old man presents with haemoptysis, dyspnoea and haematuria. Chest x-ray reveals bilateral alveolar infiltrates. Urinalysis shows protein and red cell casts.

158. A 60-year-old man presents with a chronic cough and mild haemoptysis. On examination he has digital clubbing with pain and swelling around his wrists. Chest x-ray reveals a single nodule.

159. A 30-year-old IV drug abuser presents with dyspnoea and haemoptysis. Chest x-ray is unremarkable and the ECG shows a sinus tachycardia with a mean P axis shift to the right. Blood gas shows a low $P\text{CO}_2$ and an elevated pH.

160. A 50-year-old man presents with occasional haemoptysis and chronic productive cough. He has a history of recurrent pneumonia. Chest x-ray reveals peribronchial fibrosis.

Theme: Causes of proteinuria

Options

    A Alport's syndrome
    B Minimal change disease
    C Lupus nephritis
    D Focal glomerulosclerosis
    E Membranoproliferative glomerulonephritis
    F Mesangial proliferative glomerulonephritis
    G Membranous glomerulonephritis
    H Idiopathic crescenteric glomerulonephritis
    I   Diabetic nephropathy
    J Henoch–Schönlein purpura
    K Goodpasture's syndrome
    L Postinfectious glomerulonephritis

For each case below, choose the SINGLE most likely cause from the above list of options. Each option may be used once, more than once, or not at all.

161. A 40-year-old man presents with proteinuria, haematuria and progressive renal failure. He is noted to have a high frequency sensorineural hearing loss. He has a sister who was noted to have microscopic haematuria but is asymptomatic.

162. A 7-year-old boy presents with generalised oedema and proteinuria. Electron microscopy reveals fusion of the epithelial foot processes and normal-appearing capillary and basement membranes.

163. A 30-year-old heroin addict presents with hypertension, oedema, oliguria and is noted to have heavy proteinuria. Renal biopsy specimen reveals loss of glomerular cellularity and collapse of capillary loops. Adhesions between portions of the glomerular tuft and Bowman's capsule are also seen.

164. A 12-year-old boy presents with sudden onset of haematuria and oedema. Further investigations reveal proteinuria and hypocomplementaemia (C3). Subepithelial humps and foot process fusion are seen by electron microscopy.

165. A 4-year-old boy presents with a faint leg rash, bloody diarrhoea and oliguria. Further investigations reveal heavy proteinuria and an elevated serum IgA.

Options

A HLA-B27 antigen
B Bone scan
C Antibody to ds DNA
D Anti-nucleolus antibody
E Rheumatoid factor
F HLA-DR4 antigen
G Synovial fluid analysis with polarised-light microscopy
H X-ray
I   Anti-centromere antibody
J   Anti-Jo-1 antibody
K Serum uric acid
L Anti-Ro antibody

For each case below, choose the SINGLE most discriminating investigation from the above list of options. Each option may be used once, more than once, or not at all.

166. A 60-year-old man with alcohol dependence presents with a hot, swollen first metatarsophalangeal joint and a lesion on the rim of his left pinna.

167. A 65-year-old woman with a history of hypothyroidism presents with a warm, painful swollen knee with effusion. Serum calcium is normal. X-ray reveals chondrocalcinosis.

168. A 40-year-old woman presents with flexion deformities of her fingers. She has soft tissue swelling of her digits. She also complains of difficulty swallowing and is noted to have a beaked nose and facial telangiectasia.

168. A 30-year-old woman presents with painful digits worse in the cold and difficulty swallowing. She is noted to have tapered fingers and a fixed facial expression with facial telangiectasia. X-ray reveals calcium around her fingers.

170. A 20-year-old woman presents with dry eyes, arthralgia, dysphagia and Raynaud's phenomenon.

Theme: Causes of diarrhoea

Options

    A Campylobacter infection
    B Viral gastroenteritis
    C Ulcerative colitis
    D Crohn's disease
    E Laxative abuse
    F Pseudomembranous colitis
    G Shigella infection
    H Cryptosporidiosis infection
    J Salmonellosis
    K Irritable bowel syndrome
    L *Clostridium perfringens* infection
    M *Escherichia coli* infection

For each presentation below, choose the SINGLE most likely cause from the above list of options. Each option may be used once, more than once, or not at all.

171. A 30-year-old man with AIDS presents with profuse watery diarrhoea. Oocysts are detected in the stool.

172. A 25-year-old man presents with fever, bloody diarrhoea and cramping for several weeks that does not resolve with antibiotic therapy. Proctosigmoidoscopy reveals red, raw mucosa and pseudopolyps.

173. A 60-year-old man presents with fever, watery diarrhoea and crampy abdominal pain. He had completed antibiotic therapy for osteomyelitis a month ago. Proctosigmoidoscopy reveals yellowish-white plaques on the mucosa.

174. A 20-year-old man recently back from holiday in the Far East presents with abrupt onset of severe diarrhoea. The diarrhoea is self-limiting and lasts only 3 days.

175. A 20-year-old female presents with chronic watery diarrhoea. She is emaciated. Stool electrolyte studies show an osmotic gap. Blood tests reveal hypokalaemia.

Theme: Treatment of medical emergencies

Options

    A Intramuscular epinephrine (adrenaline)
    B Emergency tracheostomy
    C Urgent endotracheal intubation
    D Type and crossmatch blood
    E Transfuse O negative blood and apply external fixator
    F Transfer to burn unit
    G Tetanus prophylaxis
    H Intravenous antibiotics
    I   Intravenous dexamethasone
    J Oxygen and nebulised salbutamol
    K Take patient straight to theatre

For each case below, choose the SINGLE most appropriate treatment from the above list of options. Each option may be used once, more than once, or not at all.

176. A 40-year-old pedestrian, struck by a speeding car, is brought into Casualty wearing a pneumatic antishock garment for an extensive open avulsion injury to her pelvis. She is intubated with fluids running via two large-bore intravenous cannulas. Blood pressure is 120/60. The pelvis is grossly distorted.

177. A 10-year-old boy burn victim is brought into Casualty with worsening stridor. A face mask with 100% oxygen is covering his face, but his oxygen saturation continues to fall. His midface and mouth have been severely burned.

178. A 4-year-old girl presents with fever, stridor and dyspnoea. She is sitting forward, drooling saliva. She has no history of asthma. She is becoming more distressed.

179. An 18-year-old man presents with fever, trismus and stridor. His breathing becomes laboured with use of accessory muscles. He becomes cyanotic. He initially presented to his GP with a sore throat a few days ago.

180. A 13-year-old known asthmatic presents with severe wheezing and a respiratory rate of 30. Pulse rate is 120.

Theme: Causes of poisoning

Options

    A Lead
    B Paracetamol
    C Salicylate
    D Arsenic
    E Ethanol
    F Mercury
    G Cyanide
    H Carbon monoxide
    I Organophosphate insecticides
    J Paraquat
    K Ethylene glycol
    L Methanol

For each case below, choose the SINGLE most likely cause from the above list of options. Each option may be used once, more than once, or not at all.

181. A 4-year-old child presents with anorexia, nausea and vomiting. On examination he has a blue line on the gums and is noted to have a foot drop. Blood test reveals anaemia.

182. A 16-year-old girl presents with weakness, excessive salivation, vomiting, abdominal pain and diarrhoea. There is 'raindrop' pigmentation of the skin. Diagnosis is made from nail clippings.

183. A 40-year-old farmer presents with acute shortness of breath and headache. His skin is red in colour, and he smells of bitter almonds.

184. A 40-year-old woman complains of headache and memory impairment following the installation of a gas fireplace. Her skin colour is pink.

185. A 50-year-old farmer presents with nausea, vomiting, hypersalivation and bronchospasm.

Theme: Treatment of diabetic complications

Options

    A Insulin sliding scale, heparin and 0.9% normal saline
    B Insulin sliding scale, heparin and 0.45% normal saline
    C Insulin sliding scale, 0.9% normal saline and potassium replacement
    D Insulin sliding scale, 0.45% normal saline and potassium replacement
    E 50 ml 50% dextrose IV
    F Sugary drink
    G Chest x-ray
    H Measure C-peptide levels

For each case below, choose the SINGLE most appropriate treatment from the above list of options. Each option may be used once, more than once, or not at all.

186. A 67-year-old man is noted to have a glucose of 37 mmol/L and a Na of 163 mmol/L. He has no prior history of diabetes and has been on intravenous fluids for a week. His other medications include IV cefuroxime, metronidazole, and dexamethasone.

187. A 60-year-old man is brought into Accident and Emergency in an unconscious state. Serum glucose is 35 mmol/L. Arterial blood gas shows pH 7.2 and a $Paco_2$ 2. Serum Na is 140, K is 3.0, Cl is 100 and the HCO_3 is 5 mmol/L.

188. A 40-year-old actor with a history of diabetes is started on propranolol for stage-fright. He collapses after a day shooting. He has not changed his insulin regime. Serum glucose is 1.5 mmol/L.

189. A 50-year-old man with a history of diabetes presents in a coma. He is febrile with diminished breath sounds on auscultation. He has warm extremities. Serum glucose is 20 mmol. The white count is 22 with increased neutrophils.

190. A 50-year-old woman presents with tachycardia, sweating and agitation. Her husband has diabetes. She has a history of Munchausen's syndrome.

Theme: Diagnosis of cardiovascular diseases

Options

A Angina pectoralis
B Aortic stenosis
C Tricuspid regurgitation
D Aortic regurgitation
E Myocardial infarction
F Acute pericarditis
G Hypertrophic obstructive cardiomyopathy
I Mitral regurgitation
J Congestive cardiomyopathy
K Mitral stenosis
L Restrictive cardiomyopathy
M Constrictive pericarditis
N Dressler's syndrome

For each case below, choose the SINGLE most likely diagnosis from the above list of options. Each option may be used once, more than once, or not at all.

191. A 40-year-old man presents with inspiratory chest pain 2 months after a heart attack. On examination a friction rub is heard in both systole and diastole. ECG shows ST elevation throughout.

192. A 35-year-old IV drug abuser presents with right upper quadrant abdominal pain. On examination there is peripheral oedema, ascites and a pulsatile liver. On auscultation there is a holosystolic murmur along the left sternal border.

193. A 30-year-old man presents with chest pain and feeling faint. On examination there is a pansystolic murmur and a fourth heart sound. ECG shows left ventricular hypertrophy. Echo shows septal hypertrophy and abnormal mitral valve motion.

194. A 40-year-old woman with Marfan's syndrome presents with shortness of breath, fainting spells and pounding of the heart. On examination there is capillary pulsation in the nail bed and pistol-shot femoral pulses. On auscultation there is a high-pitched diastolic murmur heard best at the lower left sternal edge.

195. A 40-year-old man presents after fainting during a work-out in the gym. On auscultation there is a harsh mid-systolic crescendo-decrescendo systolic murmur in the aortic area radiating to the carotids.

Theme: Treatment of cardiac arrythmias

Options

    A Atropine 1 mg IV push
    B Precordial thump
    C CPR until a defibrillator is present
    D CPR, epinephrine (adrenaline) 1 : 1000 IV push
    E Transvenous pacemaker
    F Defibrillate at 200 J
    G External pacemaker
    H Oxygen 4 L/min
    I Lidocaine (lignocaine) IV
    J Morphine IM

For each patient below, choose the SINGLE most appropriate treatment from the above list of options. Each option may be used once, more than once, or not at all.

196. A 60-year-old man presents with chest pain and shortness of breath. ECG shows sinus bradycardia of 45 beats/min.

197. A 55-year-old woman is noted to have a slow heart rate. She is asymptomatic. ECG shows no relation between atrial and ventricular rhythm. The ventricular rhythm is 40 beats/min. The QRS complex is wide.

198. A 60-year-old man collapses in the street. The event is unwitnessed. He has no pulse.

199. A 30-year-old man involved in a high speed RTA is found unconscious at the scene. He is breathing spontaneously. In Accident and Emergency, the ECG monitor now shows an irregular rhythm and no P, QRS, ST or T waves. The rate is rapid.

200. A 50-year-old man presents to Casualty with severe chest pain. He has a history of angina. The pain is not relieved with GTN. BP is 120/70 with a pulse rate of 100. ECG shows regular sinus rhythm.

Answers to Medicine SBAs/BOFs

1. E

2. D. The common peroneal nerve may be injured at the neck of the fibula.

3. D

4. A

5. C. The rash is erysipelas.

6. A

7. C

8. C

9. A

10. C

11. E

12. E

13. B

14. D

15. B

16. E

17. E. The patient has syphilis.

18. B. The patient has a subdural haematoma.

19. C. The patient has Kaposi's sarcoma.

20. C

21. E

22. B

23. B

24. B

25. A

26. D

27. A

28. D

29. A

30. B

31. A

32. A

33. A

34. B

35. C

36. C

37. C. Grey–Turner's sign is associated with acute pancreatitis.

38. E

39. D

40. C

41. C

42. C

43. C

44. C

45. C

46. C

47. B

48. E. The patient has vitamin B_{12} deficiency.

49. B. Seminomas are radiosensitive.

50. B

51. D

52. A

53. D. Also known as lateral medullary syndrome.

54. C

55. D

56. C

57. C. ACE inhibitors should be avoided in silent atherosclerosis, in particular renal artery stenosis, and may precipitate acute renal failure if administered.

58. E

59. E

60. C

61. B

62. D

63. D

64. A

65. C

66. A

67. D

68. C

69. B

70. D

71. A. The patient has infective endocarditis.

72. A

73. C

74. C

75. D

76. D

77. A

78. B. The patient has Hodgkin's disease.

79. C

80. B

81. A

82. B. The patient has prerenal failure.

83. E

84. C

85. E. This is a case of gout precipitated by thiazide diuretics.

86. D. Seizures may be associated with pethidine.

87. D

88. E

89. C

90. D

91. A

92. B

93. B

94. D

95. A

96. B

97. D

98. E

99. E. Heparin may be associated with hyperkalaemia and not hypokalaemia.

100. D

101. B

102. C

103. A

104. C

105. A

106. B

107. B

108. B

109. B

110. A

111. C

112. B

113. E

114. C

115. D

116. B

117. B

118. E

119. E

120. B

121. E. Bone metastases are usually associated with low albumin and increased alkaline phosphatase.

122. E

123. B

124. B

125. C

126. A

127. B

128. B. ECG changes in cor pulmonale include p pulmonale, RAD, RVH and inverted T waves in V1–4. The chest x-ray and ABG may be normal. Lung function tests will show air-flow restriction.

129. A

130. C

131. D

132. C

133. D

134. A

135. C

136. B

137. A

138. B. Needle cricothyroidotomy may be necessary as an emergency procedure in casualty. The leading cause of death from glandular fever (infectious mononucleosis) is failed endotracheal intubation! Bear in mind that the patient has jaw trismus! Needle cricothyroidotomy will buy time for tracheostomy by an ENT surgeon in theatre.

139. A

140. B

141. C

142. C

143. B

144. B

145. A. *Neisseria gonorrhoea* affects columnar epithelium. The vagina is composed of squamous epithelium. This explains why the endocervix and not the vagina is swabbed for the presence of the organism.

146. B

147. D

148. B

149. E

150. A

151. A. The patient exhibits Charcot's triad.

152. B

153. C. Penicillamine is a form of treatment for rheumatoid arthritis.

154. C

155. B

156. B. This patient has uraemia.

157. D. Cystic fibrosis is associated with chronic infection with *Pseudomonas aeruginosa*.

158. B

159. C

160. C

161. B

162. B. The palmar macules described are Janeway lesions.

163. E

164. B

165. D

166. E

167. A

168. E

169. D

170. E

171. A

172. A

173. D. Peptic ulcer disease is associated with hypercalcaemia not hypocalcaemia.

174. B

175. A

176. A. Erythromycin is the recommended antibiotic for legionella.

177. A. Hypothyroidism and not hyperthyroidism is associated with impotence.

178. A

179. B

180. E

181. C

182. E

183. D

184. C

185. B

186. C. This investigation is highly diagnostic for parathyroid adenomas and for pre-operative localisation of the parathyroid glands.

187. B

188. D

189. E

190. B. TCA overdose is associated with fits, arrhythmias, urinary retention and pupillary dilation. Barbiturate poisoning is also associated with pupillary dilation but not with arrhythmias.

191. A

192. B

193. C

194. D

195. D

196. A

197. B

198. A

199. D

200. B

201. C. Pulseless ventricular tachycardia is a shockable rhythm.

202. B

203. E. Option D Eaton–Lambert syndrome is associated with small-cell carcinoma of the bronchus.

204. B

205. D. Caffeine intoxication and not withdrawal may mimic panic disorder.

206. E

207. D. Patients with bulimia have irregular periods. Patients with anorexia have no periods.

208. C

209. D

210. C

211. C

212. D. The boy's anti-nuclear antibodies are positive which is associated with the development of iritis and may lead ultimately to blindness.

213. D

214. A

215. E. Post-splenectomy may be associated with early thrombocytosis.

216. A. The patient needs to be sedated prior to synchronised cardioversion and expert help is required

217. A

218. C

219. B

220. A. As the patient is asymptomatic, no treatment is advised at this time.

221. C

222. B

223. C

224. B. This patient has a partial III palsy as the pupils are spared.

225. C

226. B

227. D

228. B

229. B. Digoxin toxicity may be precipitated by hypokalaemia. The ECG changes are consistent with hypokalaemia.

230. C

231. C

232. C

233. B

234. E

235. B

236. E

237. C

238. C

239. B. Although technically the patient has veno-occlusive disease secondary to bush tea (Jamaican herbal tea) containing pyrrolidizine alkaloids. This condition resembles Budd–Chiari syndrome.

240. A

241. B. Cannabis is detectable in urine for up to 27 days with chronic use and for years if a sample of hair is analysed.

242. D. The mass is most likely an ovarian tumour.

243. B

244. C

245. E

246. A

247. C. FNA is less invasive than a trucut biopsy. FNA can also be used to distinguish between a cystic and a solid lump.

248. C

249. E. *Streptococcus pneumoniae* meningitis is more common among the elderly.

250. C

251. B

252. A

253. C

254. C

255. C

256. D. Ankylosing spondylitis is associated with both aortic regurgitation and pulmonary fibrosis. X-ray of the spine should show squaring of the vertebrae and a characteristic bamboo spine.

257. C

258. A

259. B

260. D. Enalapril is an ACE inhibitor.

261. A

262. A. Pleural plaques are associated with asbestosis. Lung function tests will confirm restrictive lung disease.

263. D. There is no cure, however corticosteroids are offered. Asbestosis is a risk factor for bronchial carcinoma.

264. D. Heminevrin (chlormethiazole) is no longer recommended for alcohol detoxification as it has been associated with fatalities when taken concurrently with alcohol. Acamprosate may be offered if a patient requests help in alcohol abstinence following detoxification. Diazepam is the drug of choice for alcohol detoxification.

265. E

266. E. This is standard advice for epilepsy.

267. D

268. E

269. E. Triple therapy is only indicated after confirmation of the presence of *Helicobacter pylori*.

270. A

271. B

272. C

273. A

274. A

275. C

276. E. Hypoglycaemia is associated with transient loss of consciousness and is reversed immediately with 50% dextrose, 50 ml IV.

277. C

278. C

279. D

280. B

281. B

282. B. In a dehydrated patient, early pneumonia will not show up on chest x-ray! Following rehydration, the pulmonary infiltrate will be more apparent.

283. E

284. A. This patient has signs of impending uncal herniation. Seek a neurosurgical consult for possible burr holes.

285. B. This patient has metastatic breast carcinoma and presents in hypercalcaemic coma.

286. C

287. A

288. A

289. A

290. E

291. E

292. C

293. D. This is a feature of ulcerative colitis.

294. E. Platelet count should be checked regularly as heparin may produce an idiosyncratic reaction.

295. E. Subcutaneous fragmin bd is used as prophylaxis and not treatment of DVT.

296. A

297. A

298. D

299. A

300. A

Answers to Medicine EMQs

1. H

2. G. Solar keratosis is a premalignant condition.

3. F

4. C. Café au lait patches are associated with neurofibromatosis.

5. B. Acral lentiginous melanoma is often mistaken for subungual haematoma or chronic paronychia. The condition can also present as expanding areas of brown or black pigmentation on the palms or soles.

6. A

7. J

8. E

9. B

10. F

11. K. This patient has Addison's disease.

12. G. This patient presents with classic signs and symptoms of hypothyroidism.

13. A. Viable protozoon cysts are ingested in contaminated food.

14. H. This patient presents with pancreatic cancer. Sudden onset in an elderly patient may be suspicious for pancreatic cancer.

15. I. Barium swallow followed by upper GI endoscopy are needed to exclude oesophageal pathology.

16. H. Infectious mononucleosis is associated with hepatitis.

17. I. This is a case of subacute bacterial endocarditis.

18. D. Unilateral enlargement of the tonsil may either be associated with quinsy, lymphoma or carcinoma. Fluctuating fever and the absence of pain suggest a diagnosis of lymphoma.

19. J. Typical features of sarcoidosis for which the Kveim test is diagnostic.

20. G. Scrofula is a sign of tuberculosis for which the Mantoux text is diagnostic.

21. H. Children under 5 are at risk, as they do not develop specific antibodies against *Haemophilus influenzae* until after the age of 5.

22. D. Tuberculous meningitis.

23. A. Meningococcal meningitis.

24. K. Viral meningitis.

25. I. Oral rifampicin is the recognised prophylactic treatment for close contacts.

26. C

27. J

28. D. Pernicious anaemia is also associated with antibodies to parietal cells.

29. A. Alcoholism is more associated with vitamin B_1 and folate deficiency. Here gastrectomy is the aetiology of the vitamin B_{12} deficiency.

30. I. Heinz bodies are associated with G6PDD.

31. A

32. D

33. C

34. B

35. C

36. K. Pretibial myxoedema is associated with hyperthyroidism.

37. H. Necrobiosis lipoidica is associated with diabetes mellitus.

38. I. Dermatitis herpetiformis is associated with coeliac disease.

39. F. Erythema multiforme may be associated with Stevens–Johnson syndrome.

40. B

41. H

42. E

43. G

44. C

45. B

46. L

47. K

48. E

49. C

50. D

51. K. The T wave changes in V5 and V6 suggest a lateral component to the inferior MI.

52. C. Atrial fibrillation may be associated with hyperthyroidism.

53. F

54. H. Hypokalaemia is a recognised complication of diuretic use.

55. G

56. B

57. G

58. A

59. C

60. F

61. C

62. E

63. B

64. I

65. G

66. C. Cold haemagglutinins are associated with 50% of untreated *Mycoplasma pneumoniae* infection and a titre of 1 : 64 supports the diagnosis.

67. J

68. A

69. B

70. F

71. K. Weight loss and salt restriction are advocated initially.

72. A

73. B. As this patient is an asthmatic, beta-blocker therapy is contraindicated.

74. I

75. E

76. J. Leptospirosis (Weil's disease) is a spirochaete transmitted in water infected by rat urine.

77. F. Kala-azar or leishmaniasis is spread through the lymphatics via a cutaneous lesion.

78. G

79. B

80. I. Felty's syndrome is the triad of rheumatoid arthritis, splenomegaly and leucopenia.

81. K

82. F

83. B

84. A

85. D

86. A. Hypokalaemia is associated with the use of loop diuretics.

87. H. Convex elevation is suggestive of MI. Here the elevation is concave which is associated with pericarditis.

88. G. A diagnosis of inferior MI requires a Q wave in lead II also.

89. C. Hypocalcaemia is a recognised complication of thyroidectomy.

90. J. Classic for myxoedema.

91. J. Anaphylaxis is treated with a prompt injection of 1 ml of 1 : 1000 epinephrine (adrenaline) IM. This may need to be repeated.

92. C. Tension pneumothorax requires emergency needle decompression.

93. D. Cardiac tamponade requires swift needle pericardiocentesis.

94. H. This lady presents with a postoperative haematoma that needs urgent drainage as it is now compressing her trachea.

95. I. This lady is at risk for a DVT and pulmonary embolism. Occasionally the signs of DVT appear after the pulmonary embolism, which can make diagnosis difficult.

96. J. Alpha-1-antirypsin deficiency is often associated with emphysema and liver disease. Liver biopsy gives a definitive diagnosis.

97. A. Primary biliary cirrhosis is associated with hepatomegaly and a high alkaline phosphatase. Antibodies to mitochondria (AMA) are found in 95% of cases.

98. B. The classic triad for idiopathic haemochromatosis is bronze skin pigmentation, diabetes mellitus and hepato-megaly.

99. C. Kaiser–Fleischer rings are a specific sign for Wilson's dis-ease, a rare inborn error of copper metabolism that leads to a failure of copper excretion.

100. G. This combination of autoimmune disease and hepatitis is suggestive of autoimmune chronic active hepatitis.

101. H. Acute lumbar disc prolapse occurs most commonly at L5/S1.

102. J. Spinal stenosis is treated by surgical decompression.

103. A. Multiple myeloma is suggestive with a high ESR. Diagnosis is confirmed by the presence of paraprotein in the serum, Bence Jones protein in the urine and by the presence of lytic bone lesions.

104. K. Complications of Paget's disease include deafness, high-output cardiac failure and osteogenic sarcoma.

105. D. Fusion of the sacro-iliac joints is a common feature of ankylosing spondylitis.

106. F. This is a case of lower motor neuron bladder neuropathy.

107. A. Excretion urography is useful to investigate the presence of renal disease predisposing to recurrent calculi formation.

108. C. Dynamic scintigraphy is used to assess renal blood flow, and in this case it is used to establish the extent of renal per-fusion post transplantation.

109. A. An intravenous urogram will give evidence of renal func-tion in benign prostatic hypertrophy. It may show hydronephrosis, bladder enlargement with chronic retention or intravesical enlargement of the prostate.

110. A. In retroperitoneal fibrosis, excretion urography allows demonstration of obstruction to the ureter commencing at the level of the pelvic brim. Retroperitoneal fibrosis may be associated with retroperitoneal lymphoma, abdominal aortic aneurysm, and carcinoma of the bladder and colon.

111. D. Bouchard's nodes and 'poor man's gout' are signs of osteoarthritis.

112. G

113. H

114. E

115. A. Postoperative arthritis is usually due to gout.

116. H

117. E

118. F

119. J

120. I

121. B

122. C

123. F

124. I

125. G

126. L

127. J

128. K

129. H

130. F. Tricuspid regurgitation is associated with endocarditis in drug addicts.

131. A. This is transmitted via inhalation from infected parrots.

132. M

133. H

134. I

135. E

136. E. Bilateral internuclear ophthalmoplegia is almost pathognomonic for multiple sclerosis.

137. H. The Argyll Robertson pupil is almost pathognomonic for neurosyphilis. As her fasting blood glucose is normal, diabetes is excluded as a cause.

138. G

139. L

140. K. Oculomotor nerve lesion with sparing of the pupil is seen with infarction of the oculomotor nerve in diabetes. 'Sparing of the pupil' means the parasympathetic fibres, which run on the superior surface of the nerve, are spared.

141. B. Hypoparathyroidism may occur following thyroid or neck surgery.

142. K

143. I. This is a case of subdural haemorrhage. The elderly and epileptics are at risk. Head trauma may have gone unnoticed.

144. L. The purple papules are most likely Kaposi's sarcoma associated with HIV.

145. J. This is a case of hypoglycaemia. Binge drinking and poor nutrition are risk factors.

146. C

147. D. Lateral medullary syndrome is caused by occlusion of the posterior inferior cerebellar artery or one vertebral artery leading to infarction of the lateral medulla and inferior surface of the cerebellum.

148. J

149. B

150. F

151. E. Patients with cystic fibrosis are at risk of pneumonia due to *Pseudomonas aeruginosa*. Tobramycin is nephrotoxic, and therefore ciprofloxacin is a wiser choice.

152. C. *Legionella pneumophila* is transmitted through the cooling system or shower facilities associated with institutions.

153. A. Asthma may be managed initially with a salbutamol inhaler.

154. I. Cyclophosphamide is the treatment for Wegener's granulomatosis.

155. H. Farmer's lung or extrinsic allergic alveolitis is caused by inhalation of the spores of *Micropolyspora faeni*, found in mouldy hay.

156. L. Wegener's granulomatosis is confirmed by biopsy of the involved tissue.

157. G. Goodpasture's syndrome is confirmed by detecting anti-glomerular basement antibody.

158. L. Bronchial carcinoma is suggested by the presence of hypertrophic pulmonary osteoarthropathy and a solitary lung nodule. Tissue biopsy is required for a definitive diagnosis.

159. K. Pulmonary embolism and infarct can present with haemoptysis. The golden standard for diagnosis is pulmonary angiogram.

160. C. Bronchiectasis is suggested here and can be confirmed by bronchography if the patient is stable.

161. A

162. B

163. D

164. L

165. J

166. G. For the diagnosis of gout, serum uric acid is not as specific as joint fluid analysis for negatively birefringent crystals.

167. G. With pseudogout or calcium pyrophosphate arthropathy the crystals are positively birefringent.

168. D. Anti-nucleolus antibody is detected in up to 60% of patients with systemic sclerosis.

169. I. CREST syndrome, a variant of systemic sclerosis, is associated with anti-centromere antibody.

170. L. Primary Sjögren's syndrome is associated with anti-Ro antibody in 70% of cases.

171. H

172. C

173. F

174. M. Traveller's diarrhoea is associated with *Escherichia coli* infection.

175. E

176. E. This patient's chief concern will be massive blood loss. No delay should be taken to crossmatch blood. Blood should be transfused immediately. The blood pressure may be misleading as she is wearing an antishock garment. An external fixator applied by the orthopaedic surgeons will aid in pelvic fracture stabilisation and stem blood loss.

177. B. As both the nasopharynx and oropharynx are compromised, tracheostomy to achieve an airway is essential.

178. C. With *Haemophilus influenzae* epiglottitis, endotracheal intubation may be difficult. It is necessary to have an ENT surgeon at hand to perform an emergency tracheostomy if the inflamed epiglottis impedes endotracheal intubation.

179. C. Glandular fever can present as acute airway obstruction. Death from glandular fever occurs from failed endotracheal intubation. It is wise to have an ENT surgeon at hand to perform an emergency tracheostomy if necessary.

180. J. An acute asthmatic attack is treated initially with oxygen and salbutamol. If necessary IV hydrocortisone is added.

181. A. Children can acquire lead poisoning by eating lead paint chips.

182. D

183. G. Cyanide is found in many rodenticides and fertilisers and causes poisoning by inhalation or ingestion.

184. H. Carbon monoxide poisoning occurs from inadequate ventilation, in this case from the gas fireplace.

185. I. Insecticides contain inhibitors of cholinesterase and lead to the accumulation of acetylcholine.

186. B. This is the treatment for hyperglycaemic hyperosmolar non-ketotic coma.

187. C. This is the treatment for diabetic ketoacidosis. The anion gap is 38.

188. E. Propranolol has been known to induce hypoglycaemia.

189. G. This patient is most likely septic from a chest infection.

190. H. This patient has probably self-injected her husband's insulin and has factitious hypoglycaemia.

191. N. This autoimmune response to a myocardial infarction occurs weeks to months later.

192. C. In this case, infective endocarditis is the cause of the tricuspid regurgitation.

193. G. This is an autosomal dominant inherited condition of interventricular septum hypertrophy.

194. D. Marfan's syndrome is associated with aortic regurgitation.

195. B. Exertional syncope is a symptom of aortic stenosis. The systolic murmur is classically diamond-shaped.

196. A. Atropine is given to patients with symptomatic bradycardia.

197. E. Third degree AV block is managed with a transvenous pacemaker.

198. C

199. C. The patient is in ventricular fibrillation.

200. H

Surgery SBAs/BOFs

In these questions candidates must select one answer only

Questions

1. A lump is situated above and medial to the pubic tubercle and is felt on the tip of the finger when the patient coughs on scrotal invagination. The most likely diagnosis is:

    A. indirect inguinal hernia
    B. direct inguinal hernia
    C. saphena varix
    D. psoas abscess
    E. femoral hernia

2. A 50-year-old man presents with a groin lump. The lump disappears when the man lies down. He has marked varicose veins. The lump has a fluid thrill. The most likely diagnosis is:

    A. psoas abscess
    B. direct inguinal hernia
    C. saphena varix
    D. femoral artery aneurysm
    E. femoral hernia

3. A 48-year-old female complains of lower back pain radiating down the buttock, back of thigh and lateral side of leg to the foot. She also complains of altered perianal sensation and urinary incontinence. The most appropriate management would be:

    A. bedrest
    B. lumbosacral corset
    C. surgical decompression
    D. NSAIDs
    E. physiotherapy

4. A 58-year-old man presents with progressive dysphagia to liquids. Of note he has a left recurrent laryngeal nerve palsy. Appropriate management includes all of the following EXCEPT:

A. chest x-ray
B. LFTs
C. contrast swallow
D. upper GI endoscopy and biopsy
E. total parenteral nutrition

5. Acute pancreatitis may be associated with all of the following EXCEPT:

A. diabetes mellitus
B. alcoholism
C. hyperparathyroidism
D. cholelithiasis
E. corticosteroids

6. Two days after a right total hip replacement, a 60-year-old obese woman develops shortness of breath. Temperature is 37°C, blood pressure is 140/85 and respiratory rate is 35/min. On examination she has a swollen right leg. She had a left mastectomy 5 years ago for breast CA. The most likely diagnosis is:

A. lymphoedema
B. deep venous thrombosis
C. pleurisy
D. pulmonary embolus
E. haematoma

7. Appropriate measures include all of the following EXCEPT:

A. IV heparin bolus followed by heparin infusion
B. subcutaneous Fragmin
C. oxygen
D. pulmonary angiogram
E. chest x-ray

8. You are called to see a 65-year-old man for confusion while on call at night. He is climbing out of bed and shouting abuse. He is two days post DHS (dynamic hip screw) for right neck of femur fracture. You administer haloperidol IM to sedate him. On examination you find that his bladder is palpable just below the umbilicus. The next most appropriate management would be:

   A. insert a Foley catheter and send an MSU for culture and sensitivities
   B. perform a digital PR examination to palpate the prostate
   C. take blood for urea and electrolytes and prostate-specific antigen
   D. arrange prostate ultrasound
   E. administer intravenous fluids

9. On preoperative examination, you find a brown raised 1-cm lesion on a patient's calf, with irregular borders and ulceration. The next most appropriate step would be:

   A. palpate the groin for inguinal lymphadenopathy
   B. take an incisional biopsy of the lesion
   C. rebook the patient for excisional biopsy
   D. arrange for a chest x-ray
   E. notify your senior colleague

10. A 28-year-old female has been assaulted by her boyfriend. She complains of severe abdominal pain and is flailing about on the stretcher. She is on 100% oxygen by face mask. You are asked to site a venflon and take blood, but you cannot locate any peripheral veins and see needle tracks. She has dilated pupils. What would you do next?

    A. ask the anaesthetist on call to intubate the patient
    B. restrain the patient with bed sheets
    C. notify your senior colleague
    D. administer naloxone IM
    E. administer diamorphine IM

11. A 20-year-old tall man presents with marked dyspnoea and chest pain. On chest auscultation, there are no breath sounds on the left side, with hyperresonance on percussion. He has just returned from a transatlantic trip to the USA. He is on 100% oxygen and is turning blue. The most likely diagnosis is:

    A. subcutaneous emphysema
    B. tension pneumothorax
    C. pulmonary embolus
    D. *Bacillus anthracis*
    E. status asthmaticus

12. The most appropriate management would be:

    A. obtain a chest x-ray
    B. insert an intercostal chest tube and attach to underwater seal
    C. IV heparinisation
    D. administer ciprofloxacin IV
    E. administer nebuliser treatment

13. A 40-year-old man presents with haematemesis. He smells of alcohol. Following resuscitation with oxygen, intravenous fluids and blood products, what is the next most important step in management?

    A. contrast swallow
    B. upper GI series
    C. endoscopy
    D. blood for LFTs
    E. chest x-ray

14. A 30-year-old man presents with a painless swollen right testicle. Appropriate management would include all of the following EXCEPT:

    A. blood for HCG and α-fetoprotein
    B. scrotal ultrasound
    C. CT scan of the abdomen
    D. chest x-ray
    E. 12-lead ECG

15. A 36-year-old female presents with cyclical bilateral breast pain. Appropriate management after excluding sinister causes includes all of the following EXCEPT:

    A. evening primrose oil
    B. oral contraceptive pill
    C. danazol
    D. gamolenic acid
    E. bromocriptine

16. A 32-year-old woman presents with a right breast lump and right breast pain. On examination she has a tender 1-cm breast lump. The most appropriate management would be:

    A. fine needle aspiration
    B. ultrasound of the breasts
    C. mammogram
    D. trucut biopsy
    E. list for excisional biopsy

17. A 40-year-old man on high-dose steroids and azathioprine for acute exacerbation of his Crohn's disease now presents with severe upper abdominal pain and vomiting. The most likely diagnosis is:

    A. small bowel obstruction
    B. perforated peptic ulcer
    C. acute pancreatitis
    D. toxic megacolon
    E. ischaemic colitis

18. The most useful investigation would be:

    A. upright chest x-ray
    B. abdominal x-ray
    C. endoscopy
    D. contrast swallow
    E. abdominal ultrasound

19. A mammogram shows microcalcifications. The most appropriate management would be:

    A. repeat mammogram immediately
    B. breast ultrasound
    C. needle-guided breast biopsy
    D. nil
    E. repeat mammogram in I year

20. Two days after coronary artery bypass graft a 50-year-old man complains of severe abdominal pain, distension and vomiting. The serum amylase is elevated with high leukocytosis. Plain abdominal x-ray shows an ileus. The most likely diagnosis:

    A. acute mesenteric ischaemia
    B. ruptured abdominal aortic aneurysm
    C. acute pancreatitis
    D. perforated peptic ulcer
    E. small bowel obstruction

21. The definitive investigation to confirm the suspected diagnosis is:

    A. barium enema
    B. colonoscopy
    C. angiography
    D. CT scan of the abdomen
    E. abdominal ultrasound

22. A 40-year-old woman presents with a goitre. She is distressed as it is large, unsightly and causes some breathing difficulty from compression of the trachea. The least useful investigation is:

    A. chest x-ray
    B. fine needle aspiration and cytology
    C. thyroid ultrasound
    D. thyroid function tests and autoantibodies
    E. isotope radionucleotide scan

23. The most appropriate treatment for this woman would be:

    A. thyroxine
    B. propylthiouracil
    C. radioiodine
    D. carbimazole
    E. thyroidectomy

24. The following statements regarding the treatment of breast cancer are true EXCEPT:

A. Locoregional breast cancer may be treated with wide local excision + radiotherapy.
B. Locoregional breast cancer may be treated with mastectomy and radiotherapy to the flaps.
C. If the sentinel node biopsy is positive, proceed to axillary node clearance.
D. Primary chemotherapy may be used to treat inflammatory breast cancer.
E. Postmenopausal women with breast cancer and positive oestrogen receptors should be offered tamoxifen.

25. A fine needle aspirate cytology is sufficient to diagnose all of the following EXCEPT:

A. papillary thyroid carcinoma
B. follicular thyroid carcinoma
C. medullary thyroid carcinoma
D. anaplastic thyroid carcinoma
E. lymphoma

26. Complications of steroid therapy include all of the following EXCEPT:

A. avascular necrosis of the hip
B. adrenal hyperplasia
C. peptic ulceration
D. acute pancreatitis
E. osteoporosis

27. On routine preoperative examination, a 55-year-old man is found to have a pulsatile midline abdominal mass. The most useful investigation would be:

A. CT scan of the abdomen
B. digital subtraction angiography
C. ultrasound of the abdomen
D. abdominal x-ray
E. MRI scan of the abdomen

28. A 60-year-old man presents with jaundice. His urine is dark, and his stools are pale. Ultrasound of the gallbladder shows a dilated common bile duct. The most appropriate management would be:

    A. open cholecystectomy
    B. ERCP + sphincterotomy
    C. laparoscopic cholecystectomy
    D. oral ursodeoxycholate and chenodeoxycholate (bile acids)
    E. oral cholangiography

29. A parotid mass is most likely to be malignant if the following feature is present:

    A. facial nerve palsy
    B. pain
    C. recent enlargement
    D. foul duct discharge
    E. stenosed ductal meatus

30. A 30-year-old man presents with sudden onset of right-sided hearing loss and tinnitus. He denies trauma to the ear. On examination the TM is normal and the Rinne tuning fork test is negative on the right and positive on the left. The Weber tuning fork test lateralises to the left. Neurological examination is normal. The most appropriate step in management would be:

    A. admit the patient for urgent CT scan of the head
    B. arrange for MRI scan of the internal acoustic meati as an outpatient
    C. arrange for a pure tone audiogram as an outpatient
    D. arrange for tympanometry as an outpatient
    E. admit the patient for 5% CO_2 and 95% O_2 inhalation and vasodilators

31. A 65-year-old woman presents with bright red blood per rectum and weight loss. The most useful investigation would be:

    A. barium enema
    B. sigmoidoscopy
    C. colonoscopy
    D. endoscopy
    E. proctoscopy

32. A 20-year-old woman presents with a wrist laceration. To test the function of the median nerve, you ask her to:

    A. extend the thumb
    B. palmar abduct the thumb against resistance
    C. pinch paper between the thumb and index finger leading to flexion of the DIP joint
    D. extend the fingers completely and spread them apart
    E. adduct the thumb

33. Charcot's triad is:

    A. epigastric pain, jaundice and fever with rigors
    B. enlarged, tender liver, jaundice and fever with rigors
    C. palpable gallbladder, jaundice and fever with rigors
    D. fever, right upper quadrant pain and a palpable mass
    E. fever, rigors and jaundice

34. Courvoisier's Law states that 'if in the presence of jaundice the gallbladder is palpable, then the jaundice is . . .'

    A. attributable to gallstones
    B. unlikely to be due to stone
    C. likely to be due to a tumour of the head of the pancreas
    D. due to cholangitis
    E. likely to be due to carcinoma of the bile duct arising above the orgin of the cystic duct

35. What is the first diagnostic test for suspected gallstones?

    A. serum bilirubin
    B. abdominal x-ray
    C. ultrasound
    D. ERCP
    E. HIDA scan

36. The following are causes of acute pancreatitis EXCEPT:

    A. alcoholism
    B. biliary tract disease
    C. oestrogens
    D. loop diuretics
    E. mumps

37. Risk factors for DVT include all of the following EXCEPT:

    A. total hip replacement
    B. caesarean section
    C. malignancy
    D. cardiac failure
    E. osteoporosis

38. What is the definitive investigation for DVT?

    A. duplex scanning
    B. Doppler ultrasound
    C. venous plethysmography
    D. venography
    E. V/Q scan

39. What is the most common cause of postoperative renal failure?

    A. pre-existing renal disease
    B. hypertension
    C. renal artery stenosis
    D. diabetes mellitus
    E. hypovolaemia

40. A 60-year-old man has a temperature of 38.5°C without rigors 24 hours postoperatively. The most likely cause of the pyrexia is:

    A. DVT
    B. pneumonia
    C. thrombophlebitis
    D. urinary tract infection
    E. atelectasis

41. A 50-year-old man post nephrectomy 3 days ago now presents with fever and confusion. On examination there are no breath sounds in the right lung base and no bowel sounds. The most likely diagnosis is:

    A. aspiration pneumonia
    B. pulmonary embolus
    C. atelectasis
    D. pneumonia
    E. pneumothorax

42. A 55-year-old man presents with diarrhoea 3 days after abdominal aortic aneurysm repair. On examination the abdomen is distended, very tender with no active bowel sounds. The most likely diagnosis is:

    A. pseudomembranous colitis
    B. mesenteric ischaemia
    C. bowel viscus perforation
    D. Shigella dysentery
    E. faecal impaction

43. A 30-year-old cyclist is involved in a RTA. He sustains multiple injuries and undergoes open reduction and internal fixation of the right femur. On postoperative day 3 he becomes acutely short of breath. The most useful investigation is:

    A. arterial blood gas
    B. chest x-ray
    C. FBC
    D. blood cultures
    E. 12-lead ECG

44. The most likely diagnosis is:

    A. acute myocardial infarction
    B. pulmonary embolus
    C. hypovolaemia due to blood loss
    D. septicaemia
    E. chest infection

45. A 60-year-old man is diagnosed with tumour of the head of the pancreas. The patient should be offered?

    A. distal pancreatectomy
    B. pancreaticojejunostomy
    C. Whipple's procedure (pancreaticoduodenectomy)
    D. total pancreatectomy
    E. multiple drug chemotherapy with radiation

46. A 25-year-old woman presents with a right-sided neck node of 4 cm in diameter. Complete head and neck examination does not reveal the aetiology. The patient should be offered:

    A. open neck biopsy
    B. examination under anaesthesia with oesophagoscopy and bronchoscopy and blind biopsies
    C. neck ultrasound
    D. needle biopsy of the neck node
    E. MRI scan of the head and neck

47. The five 'P's' of arterial insufficiency include all of the following EXCEPT:

    A. pallor
    B. paraesthesia
    C. paralysis
    D. painless
    E. pulseless

48. McBurney's point is located:

    A. at the outer one-third of a line joining the umbilicus to the anterior superior iliac spine
    B. at the outer one-third of a line joining the umbilicus to the anterior inferior iliac spine
    C. at the inner one-third of a line joining the anterior superior iliac spine to the pubic tubercle
    D. at the inner one-third of a line joining the umbilicus to the anterior superior iliac spine
    E. at the outer one-third of a line joining the anterior superior iliac spine to the pubic tubercle

49. The borders of Hesselbach's triangle include the epigastric vessels, the edge of the rectus sheath and?

    A. Poupart's ligament (the reflected inguinal ligament)
    B. the internal oblique aponeurosis
    C. the external oblique aponeurosis
    D. transversalis fascia
    E. the conjoint tendon

50. A 45-year-old man with a history of ulcerative colitis now presents with nausea, vomiting and abdominal distension. Plain abdominal films show dilatation of the entire colon. The most likely diagnosis is:

    A. volvulus
    B. diverticular disease of the colon
    C. toxic megacolon
    D. paralytic ileus
    E. carcinoma

51. Medical management of ulcerative colitis includes all of the following EXCEPT:

    A. methylcellulose
    B. mesalazine
    C. Predsol suppository
    D. azathioprine
    D. loperamide

52. A 20-year-old man presents with a cut over the right metacarpophalangeal joint. Appropriate management includes all of the following EXCEPT:

    A. obtain a hand x-ray
    B. close with sutures using aseptic technique
    C. prescribe broad-spectrum antibiotics
    D. debride and irrigate the wound
    E. swab the wound for culture and sensitivity

53. The following statements regarding skin carcinoma are true EXCEPT:

    A. Basal cell carcinoma rarely metastasises.
    B. Squamous cell carcinoma may occur in irradiated tissue.
    C. Keratoacanthoma is premalignant.
    D. Squamous cell carcinoma grows more rapidly than basal cell carcinoma.
    E. Actinic keratoses are premalignant.

54. The different types of malignant melanoma include all of the following EXCEPT:

   A. superficial spreading
   B. lentigo maligna
   C. nodular
   D. acral lentiginous
   E. nodular sclerosing

55. A 35-year-old woman with a 2-cm breast lump and an ipsilateral mobile axillary lymph node is classified as which TNM?

   A. TI NI M0
   B. TI N2 M0
   C. T2 NI M0
   D. T2 N2 M0
   E. T3 NI M0

56. A 40-year-old woman is diagnosed with metastatic breast carcinoma. Appropriate management would include all of the following EXCEPT:

   A. chemotherapy
   B. radiotherapy for bony metastases
   C. tamoxifen
   D. ovarian ablation
   E. oral opiates

57. Complications of burns include all of the following EXCEPT:

   A. stress ulcer
   B. ARDS
   C. adynamic ileus
   D. sepsis
   E. hypoglycaemia

58. A 60-year-old woman presents with postoperative oliguria. Urine output is 10 ml per hour. The CVP line reads 10 mm Hg. On lung auscultation there are rales present. The most appropriate management would be:

A. IV fluid bolus
B. furosemide (frusemide)
C. take blood for FBC
D. obtain a portable chest x-ray
E. commence IV broad-spectrum antibiotics

59. A 30-year-old man presents with a crush injury to the right anterior leg. The leg is swollen, painful and pulseless. The most appropriate management would be:

A. fasciotomy
B. arteriogram
C. plain film x-ray of the leg
D. duplex scanning
E. commence heparin infusion

60. Indications for carotid endarterectomy include all of the following EXCEPT:

A. recurrent TIAs
B. non-stenotic atherosclerotic ulcers
C. total occlusion of the internal carotid artery
D. reduction in diameter of carotid artery by >70%
E. symptomless patients with a high-grade stenosis as prophylaxis against stroke prior to cardiac bypass surgery

61. Malignant melanoma occurring in the following sites are associated with a poorer prognosis stage for stage EXCEPT for:

A. back
B. neck
C. scalp
D. trunk
E. leg

62. A 50-year-old man presents with haematuria. MSU reveals a sterile pyuria. This is suggestive of a diagnosis of:

A. urinary calculi
B. tuberculosis
C. glomerulonephritis
D. hydronephrosis
E. neoplasm

63. A 55-year-old Caucasian man involved in a RTA is found to have blood at the urethral meatus. Management includes all of the following EXCEPT:

A. retrograde urethrogram
B. pelvic x-ray
C. suprapubic catheter
D. digital rectal examination
E. Foley catheterisation

64. Painless haematuria is most likely associated with:

A. urinary tract infection
B. bladder tumour
C. gonorrhoea
D. sickle-cell anaemia
E. renal calculi

65. A 60-year-old woman post right hemicolectomy is found to have glycosuria. This is confirmed by an elevated serum glucose. Possible causes include all of the following EXCEPT:

A. sepsis
B. pre-existing diabetes mellitus
C. parenteral nutrition
D. concurrent use of steroids
E. liver failure

66. A 70-year-old woman presents with dysphagia and regurgitation to solids. She also suffers from halitosis. There is a small lump on the left side of her neck. The most appropriate investigation is:

A. barium swallow
B. oesophagoscopy
C. neck x-ray
D. neck ultrasound
E. thyroid function tests

67. A 40-year-old woman undergoes rigid oesophagoscopy for removal of a piece of chicken bone. She now presents with severe chest pain. The most likely diagnosis is:

A. acute myocardial infarction
B. pulmonary embolus
C. oesophageal perforation
D. Boerhaave's syndrome
E. perforated peptic ulcer

68. Diagnosis is best confirmed on:

A. plain soft-tissue neck x-ray
B. 12-lead ECG
C. upright chest x-ray
D. gastrograffin swallow
E. barium swallow

69. A 20-year-old woman presents with a 5-day history of right iliac fossa pain. On examination a mass is palpated in the RIF. The abdomen is soft with active bowel sounds. Possible causes include all of the following EXCEPT:

A. ectopic pregnancy
B. appendiceal mass
C. acute appendicitis
D. ovarian cyst
E. Crohn's disease

70. Organ transplantation or grafting is offered for the following conditions EXCEPT:

A. biliary atresia
B. polycystic kidney
C. cystic fibrosis
D. primary pulmonary hypertension
E. diabetic nephropathy

71. A 70-year-old woman presents with vomiting. On examination there is a tense and tender groin lump present below and lateral to the pubic tubercle. It is not reducible and there is no cough impulse. The most likely diagnosis is:

A. strangulated indirect inguinal hernia
B. strangulated direct inguinal hernia
C. saphena varix
D. psoas abscess
E. strangulated femoral hernia

72. The most likely hernia to strangulate is:

A. umbilical
B. indirect
C. direct
D. femoral
E. obturator

73. A 50-year-old obese woman presents with pyrexia, vomiting and upper abdominal pain. On examination there is a palpable mass in the right upper quadrant. The sclerae are white. The most likely diagnosis is:

A. biliary colic
B. acute cholecystitis
C. typhoid fever
D. stone in the common bile duct
E. hiatus hernia

74. A 50-year-old man post cholecystectomy now presents with jaundice. He is apyrexial. His urine is dark and his stools are pale. The most likely diagnosis is:

A. carcinoma of the head of the pancreas
B. mucocele
C. common bile duct stone
D. primary biliary cirrhosis
E. cholangitis

75. The most useful investigation is:

A. ERCP
B. ultrasound
C. CT scan
D. IV cholangiography
E. barium meal

76. Perioperative blood transfusion is detrimental in the following condition:

    A. aortic surgery
    B. colonic carcinoma
    C. total hip replacement
    D. coronary artery bypass graft
    E. pancreatic carcinoma

77. The following are absorbable sutures EXCEPT:

    A. catgut
    B. dexon
    C. vicryl
    D. PDS
    E. prolene

78. A 60-year-old man post TURP presents with convulsions. Blood pressure is 90/50. Lab. results show hyponatraemia. The most likely complication is:

    A. clot retention
    B. haemorrhage
    C. TURP syndrome
    D. ABO incompatibility
    E. ARDS

79. Types of staging include all of the following EXCEPT:

    A. clinical
    B. radiological
    C. surgical
    D. pathological
    E. historical

80. Operative treatment for carcinoma of the splenic flexure is:

    A. right hemicolectomy
    B. transverse colectomy
    C. left hemicolectomy
    D. Hartmann's procedure
    E. total colectomy

81. Investigations in the assessment of a patient with a history of TIAs include all of the following EXCEPT:

    A. FBC
    B. 12-lead ECG
    C. CT scan of head
    D. carotid digital subtraction angiogram
    E. positron emission tomography

82. The most common cause of mechanical small bowel obstruction is:

    A. Crohn's disease
    B. hernias
    C. carcinoma
    D. adhesions
    E. gallstone ileus

83. A 50-year-old man presents with severe flank pain and haematuria. Appropriate analgaesia would be:

    A. diclofenac
    B. pethidine
    C. diamorphine
    D. co-proxamol
    E. tramadol

84. IV urogram reveals a 3-cm stone in the left renal pelvis with dilatation of the calyces. Initial treatment would be:

    A. percutaneous nephrostomy
    B. extracorporeal shock wave lithotripsy
    C. nephrolithotomy
    D. partial nephrectomy
    E. extraction using a Dormia basket

85. Appropriate prophylactic antibiotic for total hip replacement surgery would be:

    A. penicillin
    B. cefuroxime
    C. metronidazole
    D. amoxicillin
    E. flucloxacillin

86. Prophylactic antibiotic of choice for appendicectomy is:

    A. cefuroxime
    B. penicillin
    C. metronidazole
    D. vancomycin
    E. gentamicin

87. Management for splenectomy patients includes all of the following EXCEPT:

    A. preop. pneumovax
    B. preop. meningococcal vaccine
    C. preop HiB vaccine
    D. lifelong amoxicillin
    E. lifelong penicillin

88. Prophylactic antibiotic of choice for cardiac valve replacement operations is:

    A. penicillin
    B. cefuroxime
    C. co-amoxiclavulanic acid
    D. vancomycin
    E. flucloxacillin

89. Components of an audit cycle include all of the following EXCEPT:

    A. implement change
    B. select a topic
    C. observe practice
    D. compare practice with standards
    E. manage risk

90. Appropriate choice of IV fluid for resuscitation of patients with burns > 15% includes all of the following EXCEPT:

    A. hetastarch
    B. dextran
    C. gelofusine
    D. 4.5% albumin
    E. crystalloid

91. Which specific blood test should be requested for a patient with suspected DVT?

    A. FBC
    B. PT
    C. D-dimers
    D. APTT
    E. bleeding time

92. A 75-year-old man presents with urinary retention. On examination he has an enlarged prostate. Blood tests reveal a normal PSA. Appropriate management includes any of the following EXCEPT:

    A. alpha-blocker
    B. TURP
    C. anti-androgen finasteride
    D. antimuscarinic
    E. parasympathomimetic

93. A 10-year-old boy falls off his bicycle and presents with contusion of the right hand. On examination he has a swollen thenar eminence. He is tender in the anatomical snuffbox. He has weakness of the opponens pollicis and normal abductor pollicis brevis function. What is your suspected diagnosis?

    A. radial nerve palsy
    B. median nerve palsy
    C. fracture of the scaphoid
    D. Colles fracture
    E. fracture of the metacarpal bone

94. A 22-year-old IV drug abuser has injected into the anatomical snuffbox and is now unable to extend his wrist. What is his diagnosis?

    A. median nerve palsy
    B. radial nerve palsy
    C. ulnar nerve palsy
    D. scaphoid fracture
    E. Colles fracture

95. A 70-year-old man is noted to have a BP of 170/100. Prior to commencing medication, the following blood tests should be requested EXCEPT:

A. FBC
B. urea/electrolytes
C. lipids
D. TFTs
E. clotting screen

96. A 60-year-old man complains of recurrent TIAs. Initial diagnosis is made by:

A. 12-lead ECG
B. CT scan of the head
C. IV digital subtraction arteriogram of the carotids
D. duplex scan of the carotids
E. intra-arterial arch study (IADSA)

97. Complications that can occur with a tracheostomy include all of the following EXCEPT:

A. tracheal stenosis
B. posterior wall erosion
C. displaced tube
D. acquired tracheo-oesophageal fistula
E. infection with *Pseudomonas aeruginosa*

98. Complications of massive blood transfusions include all of the following EXCEPT:

A. depletion of clotting factors
B. hypocalcaemia
C. hypothermia
D. hypokalaemia
E. thrombocytopenia

99. A 60-year-old man postop. day 1 after a Hartmann's procedure presents with temperature of 40°C and a BP of 80/50. Urine output is now only 10 ml/h. The most likely diagnosis is:

A. septicaemic shock
B. cardiogenic shock
C. hypovolaemic shock
D. neurogenic shock
E. anaphylactic shock

100. Appropriate measures for this man include all of the following EXCEPT:

A. blood cultures
B. wound culture
C. start IV cephuroxime and metronidazole
D. start dopamine
E. start furosemide (frusemide)

101. A 49-year-old woman is noted to have a serum calcium of 3.2 mmol/L. She denies use of diuretics or antacids and has no family history of hypercalcaemia. She has lost a stone over the past year and complains of back pain. What is the least useful investigation?

A. serum phosphate and chloride
B. lumbar spine x-ray
C. chest x-ray
D. serum PTH
E. ultrasound scan of the parathyroid glands

102. Two weeks later, she is brought to Casualty with loss of consciousness. On examination she is noted to have a hard 3-cm breast lump. Management should include all of the following EXCEPT:

A. IV fluids
B. oxygen
C. calcitonin
D. bisphosphonates
E. tamoxifen

103. A 55-year-old woman presents with disfiguring varicose veins. She reports that her legs ache by the end of the day. Examination should include all of the following EXCEPT:

A. perform Brodie–Trendelenburg tourniquet test
B. check for cough impulse over saphenofemoral junction
C. percuss over varix
D. check peripheral pulses
E. inspect for ankle flare and eczema

104. Diagnostic investigations include all of the following EXCEPT:

A. Doppler ultrasound
B. duplex ultrasonic Doppler scan
C. varicography
D. radionucleotide venography
E. bipedal ascending plethysmography

105. A 40-year-old man presents with fever, anal pain and peri-anal inflammation. On examination you confirm a perianal abscess. The most appropriate management is:

A. EUA, I&D, ± biopsy
B. conservative treatment with metronidazole
C. bedrest and analgaesia
D. wide local excision with healing by primary suture
E. lateral sphincterotomy

106. Complications of below-knee amputations include all of the following EXCEPT:

A. neuroma
B. gas gangrene
C. osteomyelitis
D. contracture
E. phantom pain

107. Signs of inoperable breast cancer include all of the following EXCEPT:

A. peau d'orange
B. skin ulceration
C. 5-cm breast lump
D. satellite nodules
E. chest fixity

108. A 55-year-old woman with metastatic breast disease now has a pathological fracture of the right femur. The most appropriate management would be:

A. intramedullary nail
B. internal fixation with plate and screws
C. radiotherapy
D. skin traction
E. chemotherapy with CMF

109. The UK National Breast Screening Programme advises mammography every 3 years to women aged between:

    A. 40 and 65
    B. 45 and 64
    C. 50 and 64
    D. 45 and 60
    E. 35 and 59

110. Lateral neck lumps include all of the following EXCEPT:

    A. cystic hygroma
    B. branchial cyst
    C. tuberculous cervical adenitis
    D. carotid body tumour
    E. dermoid cyst

111. A 20-year-old male is brought to Casualty complaining of headache and drowsiness. On examination he has a boggy swelling over the left side of his skull. The left pupil is dilated and unresponsive to light. The most likely diagnosis is:

    A. cerebral malignancy
    B. extradural haemorrhage
    C. subdural haematoma
    D. meningitis
    E. subarachnoid haemorrhage

112. While awaiting a neurosurgical opinion, the following measures should be undertaken EXCEPT:

    A. intubation and paralysis
    B. mannitol
    C. hypocapnoeic ventilation
    D. IV broad-spectrum antibiotics
    E. high levels of oxygen inspired

113. A 17-year-old young man fell onto the crossbar of his bicycle and now complains of pain in his scrotum. On examination he has a haematoma in the perineum and scrotum and frank blood from the urethral meatus. He has the urge to urinate but cannot due to pain. He has a palpable bladder. Initial measures may include all of the following EXCEPT:

A. broad-spectrum antibiotics
B. ascending urethrography using a water-soluble contrast
C. gentle passage of a 14Fr silastic catheter per urethra
D. suprapubic cystotomy under LA
E. micturating cystogram

114. A 5-month-old baby boy is brought in by his mother. She states that he has blood and mucus in his stool. He had recently been changed from milk to solids. He has episodes of screaming and abdominal pain but appears well between attacks. The most likely diagnosis is:

A. volvulus
B. intussusception
C. gastroenteritis
D. anal fissure
E. Meckel's diverticulum

115. Of the following list of complications, total hip replacement surgery has the highest risk of:

A. death
B. DVT/PE
C. wound infection
D. urinary retention
E. sciatic nerve damage

116. A 50-year-old man presents with severe abdominal pain radiating to his back. Blood pressure is 80/40 with a pulse rate of 120. The following measures should be taken EXCEPT:

A. CT scan of the abdomen
B. 12-lead ECG
C. type and crossmatch 10 units of blood
D. give blood or plasma expanders via central line
E. crash induction of anaesthesia in the operating theatre

117. The patient is anaesthetised and on the table. You are a house officer on a busy vascular service at a DGH and the registrar informs the theatre that he is on his way but is delayed. There is no SHO on duty and the consultant is at home. The anaesthetist is unable to sustain the patient's BP. He tells you to open the patient. You decide to perform a long midline abdominal incision. You confirm a ruptured aortic aneurysm. You could buy time by all of the following EXCEPT:

A. put your hand over the hole in the aorta
B. place a clamp over the neck of the aneurysm
C. insert a large Foley catheter on an introducer through the rupture and inflate the balloon
D. place a clamp over the suprarenal aorta
E. suction the blood from the abdominal cavity

118. A 35-year-old woman presents with shortness of breath following a subtotal thyroidectomy. Likely causes include all of the following EXCEPT:

A. laryngeal oedema
B. haemorrhage into the paratracheal space
C. aspiration of vomit
D. unilateral or bilateral vocal cord palsy
E. pulmonary embolus

119. Likely complications occurring after laparoscopic cholecystectomy include all of the following EXCEPT:

A. bleeding
B. jaundice
C. biliary peritonitis
D. umbilical hernia
E. paralytic ileus

120. Initial investigations for jaundice should include all of the following EXCEPT:

A. LFTs
B. hepatitis A, B and C virology
C. urine for bilirubin and urobilinogen
D. ERCP
E. EBV and CMV serology

121. What is the best technique for managing retained common bile duct stones?

   A. ERCP and sphincterotomy
   B. endoscopic removal or destruction of stones via a T-tube tract
   C. surgical exploration
   D. electrohydraulic or laser lithotripsy
   E. irrigation down a T-tube with saline

122. A 13-year-old boy presents with fever, sore throat and right hip pain. You suspect irritable hip. Appropriate investigations include all of the following EXCEPT:

   A. FBC
   B. ESR
   C. ultrasound of hip
   D. x-ray hips
   E. bone scan

123. Appropriate management includes all of the following EXCEPT:

   A. high-dose regular paracetamol
   B. skin traction
   C. skeletal traction
   D. bed rest
   E. 24-hour observation for repeated temperature checks

124. A 22-year-old man presents with gunshot wound to the right anterior thigh. You are unable to palpate any distal pulses and the leg is cold. You are also unable to detect any pulses by Doppler ultrasound probe. The next step should be:

   A. urgent fasciotomy
   B. urgent arteriography
   C. surgical exploration
   D. x-ray of leg
   E. ascending plethysmography

125. General factors which delay healing include all of the following EXCEPT:

   A. thiamine deficiency
   B. vitamin C deficiency
   C. chemotherapy
   D. zinc deficiency
   E. uraemia

126. What is the electrolyte imbalance associated with pyloric stenosis?

A. hyperchloraemic alkalosis
B. hypochloraemic alkalosis
C. hyponatraemia
D. hyperkalaemia
E. metabolic acidosis

127. Which fluid replacement is advised for a 3-week baby boy with pyloric stenosis?

A. 0.18% dextrose 4% saline + added K
B. 0.9% saline + added K
C. Hartmann's solution
D. 5% dextrose + added K
E. 0.45% saline + added K

128. Best management for pyloric stenosis is:

A. hydrostatic reduction by barium enema
B. Ramstedt pyloromyotomy
C. duodeno-duodenostomy
D. exploratory laparotomy
E. bedrest and IV fluids

129. A 16-year-old young man presents with acute onset of severe testicular pain and swelling. There is no history of trauma. The cord is thickened and the testis is tender, hot and swollen. Management should be:

A. take urethral swabs and MSU
B. give doxycycline and ciprofloxacin
C. obtain consent and place on emergency list for possible orchidectomy and bilateral orchidopexy
D. obtain ultrasound of the testis
E. take blood for serum βHCG and α-fetoprotein

130. The surgical procedure of choice for ulcerative colitis is:

A. Hartmann's procedure
B. panproctocolectomy
C. subtotal colectomy and RIF end ileostomy
D. restorative proctocolectomy
E. split loop ileostomy

131. A 70-year-old man presents with profuse PR bleeding. He has a history of aortic valve replacement. Management may include all of the following EXCEPT:

A. colonoscopy
B. barium enema
C. radiolabelled red cell scanning
D. proctoscopy and sigmoidoscopy
E. selective mesenteric angiography

132. Treatment for angiodysplasia is:

A. right hemicolectomy
B. sigmoid colectomy
C. subtotal colectomy
D. colonoscopic laser or diathermy
E. conservative treatment with blood transfusions

133. A 65-year-old female presents with fever, vomiting and severe left lower abdominal pain. On examination she has rebound tenderness and left iliac fossa guarding. The most appropriate management would be:

A. IV broad-spectrum antibiotics and barium enema
B. flexible sigmoidoscopy
C. laparotomy and Hartmann's procedure (subtotal colectomy with ileostomy and closure of the sigmoid colon at the peritoneal reflection)
D. drainage and proximal loop colostomy
E. resection with primary anastomosis

134. The correct 5-year survival rate for Duke's stage B rectal carcinoma is:

A. 71%
B. 62%
C. 40%
D. 26.5%
E. 16.4%

135. Stigmata of liver disease include all of the following EXCEPT:

A. xanthoma
B. palmar erythema
C. gynaecomastia
D. Volkmann's contracture
E. clubbing

136. Cholangiocarcinoma is associated with which parasite?

A. *Echinococcus granulosus*
B. *Entamoeba histolytica*
C. *Schistosoma mansoni*
D. *Giardia lamblia*
E. *Clonorchis sinensis*

137. A 55-year-old homeless man presents with profuse haematemesis. He is unkempt and smells of alcohol. On examination BP is 85/50, pulse 130, and he has tender hepatomegaly and spider naevi. The most likely diagnosis is:

A. oesophageal varices
B. perforated peptic ulcer
C. Mallory–Weiss tear
D. gastric varices
E. angiodysplasia

138. Appropriate management after resuscitation includes all of the following EXCEPT:

A. arrange urgent endoscopy
B. crossmatch 6 units of blood
C. consider Sengstaken–Blakemore tube to tamponade bleed
D. administer octreotide
E. commence cimetidine

139. You are obtaining consent from a patient for partial gastrectomy and discuss the risk of dumping syndrome. Which symptom is NOT associated with this syndrome?

A. palpitations
B. diarrhoea
C. diaphoresis
D. faintness
E. nausea after eating

140. Causes of sclerosing cholangitis include all of the following EXCEPT:

A. ulcerative colitis
B. Crohn's disease
C. carcinoma
D. gallstones
E. previous biliary surgery

141. A 40-year-old woman undergoes laparoscopic cholecystectomy. This is converted to an open cholecystectomy on the table. 4 days later she develops spiking temperatures to 40°C. Chest x-ray, MSU and blood cultures are clear. White cell count is raised with predominantly neutrophils. What is the next investigation?

A. CT scan of the abdomen
B. ERCP
C. ultrasound
D abdominal x-ray
E. peritoneal tap

142. The most likely diagnosis is:

A. DVT
B. pulmonary atelectasis
C. subphrenic abscess
D. retained stones in the CBD
E. anaphylaxis

143. A 70-year-old man undergoes right total knee replacement. 12 hours postop. You are called for poor urine output of 100 ml in the last 8 hours. On examination, he is pale and dyspnoeic. His BP is 88/58 with a pulse of 110. His pulse oxymeter reads 98%. His preop. Hb was 11 g/dL. He has been on fragmin preop. and postop. You check the position of the Foley catheter. The next step is?

A. take blood for urgent FBC and crossmatch
B. insert a central line
C. perform a 12-lead ECG
D. arrange a V/Q scan
E. give boluses of IV fluids

144. Associations with gastric cancer include all of the following EXCEPT:

    A. pernicious anaemia
    B. atrophic gastritis
    C. blood group O
    D. acanthosis nigricans
    E. Sister Mary Joseph's sign

145. A 50-year-old secretary complains of tingling and numbness over the right thumb, index, middle and lateral half of the ring finger, worse at night. She also complains of weakness in holding a book. On examination there is weakness of the thumb abduction and wasting of the thenar muscles. The most likely diagnosis is:

    A. cervical spondylosis
    B. carpal tunnel syndrome
    C. multiple sclerosis
    D. rheumatoid arthritis
    E. myasthenia gravis

146. Treatment for carpal tunnel syndrome includes all of the following EXCEPT:

    A. splintage
    B. diuretics
    C. Depo-Medrone injection
    D. arthroscopic division of the flexor retinaculum
    E. NSAIDs

147. A 65-year-old man presents with low back pain and urinary incontinence. On DRE, a hard nodular prostate is palpated. Appropriate investigations include all of the following EXCEPT:

    A. prostate specific antigen
    B. isotope bone scan
    C. transrectal biopsy
    D. serum acid phosphatase
    E. CEA

148. The treatment of choice for metastatic prostate carcinoma is:

A. bilateral subcapsular orchidectomy and conservative TURP
B. long-acting luteinising hormone releasing analogues
C. chemotherapy
D. external beam radiotherapy
E. radical prostatectomy

149. Risk factors for carcinoma of the oesophagus include all of the following EXCEPT:

A. alcohol
B. smoking
C. achalasia
D. Barrett's oesophagus
E. blood group A

150. Clinical findings with pneumothorax include all of the following EXCEPT:

A. increased vocal fremitus
B. increased vocal resonance
C. raised percussion note
D. whispering pectoriloquy
E. tracheal shift to the same side

151. The following statements are true regarding blunt chest trauma EXCEPT:

A. A contused lung goes into pulmonary oedema rapidly.
B. In a normal lung, bacteria are cleared in 4 hours.
C. In a contused lung, bacteria clear in 24 hours.
D. The first two ribs are the easiest to break.
E. Fractured ribs may be repaired by wire fixation.

152. A 30-year-old woman presents with severe chest pain. She was a driver in a high-speed head-on collision. Chest x-ray shows a widened mediastinum. The most likely diagnosis is:

A. haemothorax
B. pulmonary contusion
C. mediastinal mass
D. possible ruptured aorta
E. aortic aneurysm

153. Your next step would be:

A. Arrange an urgent CT scan and then transfer the patient to a specialist centre.
B. Transfer the patient directly to a specialist centre.
C. Arrange an urgent ultrasound and then transfer the patient to a specialist centre.
D. Take the patient directly to theatre.
E. Treat the patient conservatively.

154. Investigations for potential ruptured aorta include all of the following EXCEPT:

A. arch aortogram
B. transoesophageal echo (TOE)
C. spiral CT scan
D. chest x-ray
E. MRI scan

155. The following statements regarding undescended testes are correct EXCEPT:

A. Undescended testes must be fixed by 1 year of age.
B. Ultrasound is a useful investigation in children.
C. CT scan is not indicated.
D. Most cases are retractile.
E. Surgery is offered to locate the testes via a high Jones approach and then to fix the testes.

156. The following statements regarding adenocarcinoma of the stomach are correct EXCEPT:

A. The tumour is most commonly found in the antrum.
B. Intestinal gastric CA has a better prognosis than diffuse type.
C. The investigation of choice is a double-contrast barium study + fibre-optic endoscopy.
D. Surgical laparotomy is the best method of staging this tumour.
E. Radical gastrectomy is offered for all stages of the tumour.

157. A 50-year-old man presents with dysphagia. Endoscopy and biopsies reveal adenocarcinoma at the gastric fundus. CT scan confirms hepatic metastasis. The most appropriate treatment is:

A. radical gastrectomy
B. re-establish swallowing with recanalisation with laser, intubation or bypass
C. chemotherapy with epirubicin, cisplatinum and continuous 5-FU
D. radiotherapy
E. palliative resection

158. The treatment for established ARDS is:

A. IV broad-spectrum antibiotics
B. endotracheal intubation and intermittent positive-pressure ventilation
C. respiratory physiotherapy
D. fluid replacement with plasma expanders
E. 100% oxygen by face mask

159. The following statements regarding management of burns are correct EXCEPT:

A. Full-thickness burns are established by loss of sensation to pinprick.
B. Treatment should include IV broad-spectrum antibiotics.
C. Oral opiates are used for analgaesia.
D. Fluid replacement is with purified protein fraction or albumin.
E. 2 units of blood should be given after 48 hours.

160. The most accurate investigation for diagnosing the site of an UGI bleed is:

A. double-contrast radiography
B. angiography
C. endoscopy
D. chest x-ray
E. CT scan of the chest

161. Recognised methods of controlling an UGI bleed include all of the following EXCEPT:

A. NdYAG laser with endoscopy
B. endoscopic diathermy
C. endoscopic sclerotherapy
D. balloon tamponade
E. endoscopic intubation

162. Acute osteomyelitis is most commonly associated with:

    A. *Streptococcus pneumoniae*
    B. *Haemophilus influenzae*
    C. salmonella
    D. *Staphylococcus aureus*
    E. *Streptococcus viridans*

163. A 50-year-old banker complains of retrosternal chest pain, which awakens him at 2 am in the morning. He smokes 20 cigarettes a day. He takes no medication. The most likely diagnosis is:

    A. gastric ulcer
    B. angina
    C. duodenal ulcer
    D. costochondritis
    E. oesophagitis

164. What is the recommended treatment for *Helicobacter pylori* eradication?

    A. H_2 blocker + clarithromycin + metronidazole for 1 week
    B. H_2 blocker + amoxicillin + metronidazole for 2 weeks
    C. bismuth + amoxicillin + tetracycline for 6 weeks
    D. bismuth + clarithromycin + H_2 blocker for 2 weeks
    E. bismuth + amoxicillin + metronidazole for 2 weeks

165. Indications for surgery for duodenal ulcer include all of the following EXCEPT:

    A. pyloric stenosis
    B. perforation
    C. haemorrhage
    D. lack of patient compliance with medical treatment
    E. pain

166. Preoperative management of perforated duodenal ulcer includes all of the following EXCEPT:

    A. insert a NG tube
    B. commence IV cefuroxime and metronidazole
    C. replete plasma volume with crystalloid
    D. insert a Foley catheter and maintain a urine output of 60 ml/h
    E. give diclofenac IM for analgaesia

167. A 60-year-old man on IV cefuroxime and metronidazole for acute diverticulitis, now presents with swinging pyrexia and a white cell count of $18 \times 10^9/L$. He is tender in the left iliac fossa but does not have peritoneal signs at this stage. The next step should be:

A. obtain an urgent abdominal x-ray to exclude bowel obstruction
B. obtain an upright chest x-ray to exclude perforation of a diverticulum
C. request an ultrasound to exclude pericolic abscess
D. expeditious surgery
E. continue to treat conservatively with IV antibiotics

168. A 60-year-old man presents with vomiting and severe upper abdominal pain radiating to the back. He is sitting forward. He has a history of alcoholism. On examination temperature is 39°C, BP is 90/50, and pulse is 135/min. His abdomen is rigid with generalised tenderness. Pulse oximeter reads 80% O_2 saturation. Useful blood tests include all of the following EXCEPT:

A. FBC
B. arterial blood gas
C. serum amylase
D. serum glucose
E. clotting profile

169. Chest x-ray shows a small left-sided pleural effusion. Abdominal x-ray shows absent psoas shadow. Blood results are:

WBC	$20 \times 10^9/L$
Hb	10 g/dL
Plts	$250 \times 10^9/L$
glucose	12 mmol/L
LDH	400 IU/L
AST	60 IU/L
GGT	100 IU/L
amylase	1200 IU/ml

The most likely diagnosis is:

A. perforated peptic ulcer
B. perforated gallbladder
C. acute pancreatitis
D. ruptured AAA
E. alcoholic cirrhosis

170. A 50-year-old woman returns for her mammogram results. The mammogram reveals spiculation and finely scattered microcalcification. FNAC confirms breast cancer. Further investigations for this patient include all of the following EXCEPT:

A. LFTs
B. chest x-ray
C. 12-lead ECG
D. bone scan
E. ultrasound of the liver

171. A 20-year-old man attempts suicide by drinking sulphuric acid. Management should include all of the following EXCEPT:

A. total parenteral nutrition via a central line
B. gastrostomy
C. nil by mouth
D. steroids
E. gentle dilatation with bougies after 3–4 weeks

172. Preoperative management for thyroidectomy should include:

A. ENT referral for vocal cord check
B. type and cross 2 units of blood
C. serum calcium level
D. SC Fragmin
E. CT scan of the neck

173. Indications for thyroidectomy include all of the following EXCEPT:

A. retrosternal goitre
B. unsightly goitre
C. solitary nodule
D. fear of radiation
E. myxoedema

174. A 25-year-old obese lady complains of difficulty breathing and swallowing. On examination her breathing is laboured, and her trachea is displaced. You ask her to raise her arms above her head. She develops facial congestion and stridor. The most likely diagnosis is:

   A. retrosternal goitre
   B. tension pneumothorax
   C. cervical rib
   D. oesophageal carcinoma
   E. globus pharyngeus

175. The most appropriate investigation is:

   A. plain chest x-ray + thoracic inlet view of the neck
   B. ultrasound of the neck
   C. endoscopy
   D. thyroid function tests
   E. technetium scintiscan

176. A 70-year-old man presents with left lower abdominal pain and change in bowel habits. Barium enema shows a filling defect in the sigmoid colon. The most likely diagnosis is:

   A. diverticulosis
   B. carcinoma
   C. Crohn's disease
   D. ulcerative colitis
   E. familial adenomatous polyposis

177. Signs of venous hypertension include all of the following EXCEPT:

   A. ankle flare
   B. lipodermatosclerosis
   C. varicose veins
   D. cellulitis
   E. shallow ulcers with sloping edges on the medial aspect of the leg

178. A 60-year-old man presents with acute right leg pain. On examination the leg is white, cold, desensate and pulseless. On-table angiography stops at the adductor canal. The next step is:

A. thrombolysis
B. reverse saphenous vein graft for femoral–popliteal bypass
C. primary stenting to the right iliac artery
D. dacron graft for femoral–popliteal bypass
E. reverse saphenous vein graft for femoral–posterior tibial bypass

179. A 50-year-old woman presents with pain and a cold right leg for 4 hours. On examination her pulse is irregular with a rate of 120. She has a history of mitral valve disease. The most likely diagnosis is:

A. femoral artery embolism
B. popliteal aneurysm
C. femoral aneurysm
D. intermittent claudication
E. deep venous thrombosis

180. Appropriate investigations for Crohn's disease include all of the following EXCEPT:

A. FBC
B. barium follow-through
C. colonoscopy
D. ESR, CRP
E. sigmoidoscopy

Surgery EMQs
Theme: Diagnosis of abdominal pain

Options

    A Acute appendicitis
    B Diverticular disease
    C Abdominal aortic aneurysm
    D Perforated peptic ulcer
    E Crohn's disease
    F Ulcerative colitis
    G Acute pancreatitis
    H Chronic active hepatitis
    I Acute viral hepatitis
    J Pseudo-obstruction
    K Acute cholecystitis
    L Acute diverticulitis

For each presentation below, choose the SINGLE most likely diagnosis from the above list of options. Each option may be used once, more than once, or not at all.

1. A 20-year-old man presents with colicky periumbilical pain which shifts to the RIF, fever and loss of appetite.

2. A 48-year-old man presents with severe epigastric pain radiating to the back. He is noted to have some bruising in the flanks.

3. A 42-year-old woman presents with anorexia, abdominal pain and increasing jaundice. She is asthmatic and takes methyldopa for hypertension.

4. A 50-year-old man presents with left-sided colicky iliac fossa pain, change in bowel habits and rectal bleeding. A thickened mass is palpated in the region of the sigmoid colon. Full blood count is normal.

5. A 78-year-old woman with stable angina presents with massive abdominal distension 10 days following a total hip replacement.

Theme: Diagnosis of breast diseases

Options

        A Fibroadenoma
        B Fibrocystic disease
        C Galactocoele
        D Intraductal papilloma
        E Mammary duct ectasia
        F Breast cancer
        G Cystosarcoma phylloides
        H Breast abscess
        I Fat necrosis
        J Paget's disease
        K Eczema of the nipple

For each patient below, choose the SINGLE most likely diagnosis from the above list of options. Each option may be used once, more than once, or not at all.

6. A 28-year-old female presents with a solitary 3-cm freely mobile painless nodule. She also complains of a serous nipple discharge and axillary lymphadenopathy.

7. A 36-year-old female presents with multiple and bilateral cystic breast swellings which are noted to be particularly painful and tender premenstrually. She states that during pregnancy the symptoms improved.

8. A 50-year-old woman presents with nipple discharge, nipple retraction, dilatation of ducts and chronic intraductal and periductal inflammation. The diagnosis is confirmed by breast biopsy and no further treatment is required.

9. A 50-year-old woman presents with an eczematoid appearance to her nipple and areola. It is associated with a discrete nodule that is attached to the overlying skin.

10. A 33-year-old lactating female presents with a 1-week history of a painful, erythematous breast lump and pyrexia. She has tried a course of antibiotics to no avail.

Theme: Causes of neck lumps

Options

    A Branchial cyst
    B Ludwig's angina
    C Parotitis
    D Thyroglossal cyst
    E Dermoid cyst
    F Parapharyngeal abscess
    G Thyroid swelling
    H Sialectasis
    I Laryngocoele
    J Pharyngeal pouch
    K Reactive lymphadenitis

For each presentation below, choose the SINGLE most likely cause from the above list of options. Each option may be used once, more than once, or not at all.

11. A 45-year-old clarinet player presents with a neck swelling that expands with forced expiration.

12. A 4-year-old boy presents with a small midline neck swelling which moves on swallowing. It is painless, mobile, transilluminates and fluctuates.

13. A 26-year-old man following a trip to the dentist for a toothache presents with a tender neck swelling, pyrexia and pain on swallowing. The tonsils are not inflamed.

14. A 30-year-old male presents with a 5 cm neck swelling anterior to the sternomastoid muscle on the left side in its upper third. He states that the swelling has been treated with antibiotics for infection in the past.

15. A 20-year-old man presents with a painful swelling under his jaw. On examination he has trismus and is dribbling saliva.

Theme: Treatment of postoperative pain

Options

     A Aspirin tablets
     B Diclofenac suppositories
     C Dihydrocodeine tablets
     D Patient-controlled analgaesia (PCA) with morphine
     E Intercostal nerve blocks
     F Epidural analgaesia
     G Carbamazepine
     H Paracetamol tablets
     I Diamorphine
     J Intramuscular pethidine

For each case below, choose the SINGLE most appropriate treatment from the above list of options. Each option may be used once, more than once, or not at all.

16. A 33-year-old man requires analgaesia following an exploratory laparotomy and splenectomy.

17. A 55-year-old woman with terminal metastatic breast carcinoma requires long-term analgaesia following radical mastectomy.

18. A 40-year-old man complains of phantom limb pain following a below the knee amputation.

19. A 25-year-old man underwent excision of a sebaceous cyst under local anaesthesia. He uses salbutamol inhaler on a regular basis.

20. A 60-year-old man requires analgaesia following a total thyroidectomy.

Theme: Investigation of postoperative complications

Options

A Chest x-ray
B Serum calcium
C 12-lead electrocardiogram
D Ultrasound abdomen
E Serum glucose
F Midstream specimen of urine
G Thyroid function tests
H Pulmonary angiogram
I Bladder ultrasound
J Serum haemoglobin

For each presentation below, choose the SINGLE most confirmatory investigation from the above list of options. Each option may be used once, more than once, or not at all.

21. A 55-year-old man post thyroidectomy presents with tetany. Upon tapping the preauricular region, the facial muscles begin to twitch.

22. A 50-year-old man post coronary artery bypass graft surgery presents with fever and severe epigastric pain.

23. A 70-year-old woman post dynamic hip screw for a right neck of femur fracture presents with pallor, tachycardia and hypotension. Oxygen saturation is 90%. The rest of her examination is normal.

24. A 65-year-old man 10 days post right total hip replacement presents with sudden breathlessness and collapses. On examination he is noted to have a pleural rub, increased JVP, and a swollen right leg.

25. A 35-year-old primigravida post caesarean section complains of inability to void. She denies dysuria but complains of fullness. She was treated with an epidural for analgaesia.

Theme: Investigation of abdominal pain

Options

        A Ultrasound abdomen
        B Rectal examination
        C Upper GI endoscopy
        D Barium meal
        E Sigmoidoscopy
        F Colonoscopy
        G CT scan of the abdomen
        H Kidneys, ureters and bladder (KUB) x-ray
        I Pelvic ultrasound
        J Laparoscopy
        K Erect chest x-ray

For each presentation below, choose the SINGLE most discriminating investigation from the above list of options. Each option may be used once, more than once, or not at all.

26. A 60-year-old man complains of severe colicky pain from his right flank radiating to his groin. Urinalysis reveals trace blood cells.

27. A 25-year-old woman complains of severe lower abdominal pain and increasing abdominal girth. Urine HCG is negative.

28. A 60-year-old obese man complains of severe epigastric pain radiating to his back. The pain is relieved by eating and is worse at night.

29. A 65-year-old hypertensive man presents with lower abdominal pain and back pain. An expansive abdominal mass is palpated lateral and superior to the umbilicus.

30. An 80-year-old woman suffering from rheumatoid arthritis presents with severe epigastric pain and vomiting. She also complains of shoulder tip pain.

Theme: Diagnosis of hearing problems

Options

A Presbyacusis
B Cerumen
C Acute suppurative otitis media
D Otitis externa
E Chronic secretory otitis media
F Barotrauma
G Chronic suppurative otitis media
H Dead ear
I Otosclerosis
J Temporal bone fracture
K Osteogenesis imperfecta

For each patient below, choose the SINGLE most likely diagnosis from the above list of options. Each option may be used once, more than once, or not at all.

31. A 70-year-old man presents with gradual deterioration of hearing in both ears. The Weber tuning fork test is non-lateralising and the Rinne test is positive on both sides. The tympanic membranes are intact and healthy.

32. A 60-year-old man presents with unilateral earache, diminished hearing and foul-smelling discharge. The external auditory meatus is oedematous and the canal is stenosed. The discharge is white and creamy in nature.

33. A 40-year-old woman presents with diminished hearing in the right ear. She denies earache or discharge. She is noted to have blue sclerae. The tympanic membrane is normal. The Weber tuning fork test lateralises to the right side and the Rinne is negative on the right.

34. A 4-year-old girl presents to her GP with diminished hearing noted by the school. On examination there is a bulging yellow tympanic membrane on the right alone.

35. A 70-year-old female presents with longstanding deafness in the left ear. The Weber lateralises to the right and the Rinne is negative on the left.

Theme: Diagnosis of conditions of the hand

Options

      A Volkmann's ischaemic contracture
      B Dupuytren's contracture
      C Carpal tunnel syndrome
      D Claw hand
      E Raynaud's phenomenon
      F Scleroderma
      G Rheumatoid arthritis
      H Paronychia
      I Psoriasis
      J Koilonychia
      K Glomus tumour
      L Subungual haematoma

For each presentation below, choose the SINGLE most likely diagnosis from the above list of options. Each option may be used once, more than once, or not at all.

36. A 20-year-old female presents with a painful fingertip that throbs and has kept the patient up all night. The skin at the base and side of the nail is red, tender and bulging.

37. A 30-year-old female presents with a painful fingernail. On examination there is a small purple-red spot beneath the nail. She denies trauma to the finger.

38. A 60-year-old man with acromegaly presents with pins and needles in the index and middle fingers of his right hand, worse at night.

39. A 20-year-old man presents with fingers that are permanently flexed in his right hand. However, the deformity is abolished by flexion of the wrist. He admits to trauma to his elbow recently. He also complains of pins and needles.

40. A 20-year-old female complains of intermittent pain in her fingertips. She describes the fingers undergoing colour changes from white to blue and then to red. The symptoms are worse in the winter.

Theme: Causes of haematemesis

Options

A Chronic peptic ulceration
B Gastritis
C Oesophageal varices
D Mallory–Weiss syndrome
E Carcinoma of the oesophagus
F Carcinoma of the stomach
G Oesophagitis
H Haemophilia
I Epistaxis
J Angiodysplasia
K Peutz–Jeghers' syndrome
L Ehlers–Danlos syndrome

For each case below, choose the SINGLE most likely cause from the above list of options. Each option may be used once, more than once, or not at all.

41. A 40-year-old obese man presents with projectile haematemesis after ingestion of a five-course meal and wine.

42. A 50-year-old man presents with massive haematemesis. He is noted to have freckles on his lower lips.

43. A 60-year-old alcoholic man presents with massive haematemesis and shock. He is noted to have finger clubbing and ascites.

44. A 70-year-old man with chronic hoarseness presents with retrosternal chest pain and haematemesis. He has a history of achalasia and has lost one stone in weight.

45. A 65-year-old man presents with haematemesis. He is noted to have an enlarged left supraclavicular node, ascites and anaemia.

Theme: Causes of abdominal masses

Options

    A Psoas abscess
    B Appendicitis
    C Tuberculosis
    D Crohn's disease
    E Diverticulitis
    F Carcinoma in the sigmoid colon
    G Carcinoma of the caecum
    H Obstruction of the common bile duct by a calculus
    I Carcinoma of the pancreas
    J Ovarian cyst
    K Mesenteric cyst

For each case below, choose the SINGLE most likely cause from the above list of options. Each option may be used once, more than once, or not at all.

46. A 40-year-old man presents with fever, painless jaundice and a palpable gallbladder.

47. A 30-year-old woman presents with colicky abdominal pain and distension. On examination a smooth, mobile, spherical mass is palpated in the centre of her abdomen. A fluid thrill is elicited, and the mass is dull to percussion.

48. A 20-year-old man presents with fever, abdominal and back pain and a mass in the right iliac fossa. The swelling is soft, tender, dull and compressible. It extends below the groin. He denies nausea, vomiting or diarrhoea.

49. A 50-year-old man presents with a dull ache in the right iliac fossa and diarrhoea. A freely mobile mass is palpated in the right iliac fossa. The rectum is normal and the faeces contain blood.

50. A 55-year-old man presents with severe left iliac fossa pain, nausea and chronic constipation. A tender, sausage-shaped mass is palpated in the left iliac fossa.

Theme: Causes of shock

Options

A Pulmonary embolism
B Myocardial ischaemia
C Cardiac tamponade
D Trauma
E Burns
F Sepsis
G Anaphylaxis
H Major surgery
I Ruptured aortic aneurysm
J Ectopic pregnancy
K Addisonian crisis
L Hypothyroidism
M Acute pancreatitis

For each patient below, choose the SINGLE most likely cause from the above list of options. Each option may be used once, more than once, or not at all.

51. A 50-year-old man arrives at Casualty in shock. BP is 80/50. The heart sounds are muffled. The JVP increases with inspiration.

52. A 30-year-old woman presents to Casualty in respiratory distress and shock. She is noted to have stridor. Her lips are swollen and blue.

53. A 55-year-old man presents to Casualty with severe abdominal pain, vomiting and shock. The pain is in the upper abdomen and radiates to the back. He takes diuretics. The abdomen is rigid, and the x-ray shows absent psoas shadow.

54. A 40-year-old woman presents to Casualty in shock with continuous abdominal pain radiating to her back. The abdomen is rigid with an expansile abdominal mass.

55. A 35-year-old woman presents to Casualty in shock with a BP of 80/50 and tachycardia. She is confused and weak. Her husband states, that she forgot to take her prednisolone tablets with her on holiday and has missed several doses.

Theme: Treatment of fractures and dislocations

Options

        A Kocher's method
        B AO cannulated screws
        C Bedrest
        D Open reduction and Kirschner wire
        E Buddy strapping
        F Reconstructive surgery with internal graft or implant augmentation
        G Physiotherapy for strengthening exercises
        H Austin Moore hemiarthroplasty
        I   Dynamic hip screw
        J   Total hip replacement
        K Open reduction and internal fixation

For each of the cases below, choose the SINGLE most appropriate treatment from the above list of options. Each option may be used once, more than once, or not at all.

56. A 50-year-old fit man presents with a right hip fracture. On x-ray the fracture line is subcapital.

57. A 20-year-old athlete twists his knee on holiday while skiing. On examination he has a positive drawer sign with the tibia sliding anteriorly.

58. A 70-year-old woman presents with a left hip fracture. On x-ray the fracture line is intertrochanteric.

59. A 40-year-old woman sprains her wrist. She complains of persistent pain and tenderness over the dorsum distal to Lister's tubercle. X-rays show a large gap between the scaphoid and the lunate. In the lateral view, the lunate is tilted dorsally and the scaphoid anteriorly.

60. A 30-year-old basketball player presents with severe pain in his shoulder. He is holding his arm with the opposite hand. He explains that he fell on an outstretched hand. The x-ray shows overlapping shadows of the humeral head and glenoid fossa, with the head lying below and medial to the socket. There is also a fracture of the neck of the humerus.

Theme: Management of traumatic injuries

Options

- A Peritoneal lavage
- B Observation and angiography
- C Closed thoracostomy-tube drainage
- D Pressure dressing
- E Cricothyroidotomy
- F Nasogastric tube suction and observation
- G Surgical repair of the flexor digitorum superficialis tendon
- H Surgical repair of the flexor digitorum profundus tendon
- I Urgent surgical exploration
- J Debridement and repair
- K Endotracheal intubation
- L Needle pericardiocentesis
- M Fasciotomy

For each case below, choose the SINGLE most appropriate management from the above list of options. Each option may be used once, more than once, or not at all.

61. A 23-year-old man presents to Accident and Emergency having been stabbed in the neck. He complains of difficulty swallowing and talking. He has no stridor. On examination there is a small penetrating wound with diffuse neck swelling.

62. A 12-year-old boy presents with a hand injury sustained while attempting to catch a ball. On examination he is unable to bend the tip of his right middle finger.

63. A 35-year-old woman is brought into Accident and Emergency acutely short of breath. Respiratory rate is 50/min. She was involved in a road traffic accident. There are no breath sounds auscultated on the left. The trachea is deviated to the right.

64. An 18-year-old man sustains a stab wound to the right thigh. On examination there is a large haematoma over the thigh and weak distal pulses. He is unable to move his foot and complains of pins and needles in his foot.

65. A 30-year-old woman involved in a head-on car collision presents with diffuse abdominal pain. Upright chest x-ray shows elevation of the diaphragm with a stomach gas bubble in the left lower lung field.

Theme: Diagnosis of gastrointestinal conditions

Options

A Hepatoma
B Oesophageal varices
C Mallory–Weiss tear
D Perforated peptic ulcer
E Fractured rib
F Haematoma of the rectus sheath
G Umbilical hernia
H Sigmoid volvulus
I Splenic rupture
J Pancreatic pseudocyst
K Divarication of the recti
L Acute pancreatitis

For each case below, choose the SINGLE most likely diagnosis from the above list of options. Each option may be used once, more than once, or not at all.

66. A 50-year-old alcoholic man presents with nausea, vomiting and epigastric pain. On examination there is a palpable epigastric mass. The amylase is raised. CT scan of the abdomen shows a round well-circumscribed mass in the epigastrium.

67. A 40-year-old multiparous woman presents with a midline abdominal mass. The mass is non-tender and appears when she is straining. On examination the midline mass is visible when she raises her head off the examining bed.

68. A 19-year-old man presents with sudden severe upper abdominal pain after being tackled during rugby practice. He was recently diagnosed with glandular fever.

69. A 7-year-old girl presents with spontaneous massive haematemesis.

70. A 55-year-old male alcoholic presents with vomiting 800 ml of blood. Blood pressure is 80/50 with a pulse rate of 120. Ascites is noted.

Theme: Management of postoperative complications

Options

A Intravenous dantrolene sodium
B Intravenous calcium gluconate
C Blood transfusion
D Blood cultures
E Obtain chest x-ray
F Midstream urine collection for culture
G Intravenous broad-spectrum antibiotics
H Insulin in dextrose
I Foley catheterisation
J Obtain abdominal x-ray
K Check full blood count

For each case below, choose the SINGLE most appropriate management option from the above list of options. Each option may be used once, more than once, or not at all.

71. A 30-year-old female post appendicectomy develops high fever of 42°C, hypotension, and mottled cyanosis in the recovery room. She received halothane inhalation gas in surgery. She was noted to have trismus during intubation.

72. A 40-year-old man complains of circumoral numbness following thyroidectomy. Tapping over his preauricular regon elicits facial twitching.

73. A 50-year-old man post nephrectomy becomes febrile, confused, tachypnoeic and tachycardic. He was recently advanced to a soft diet. There are no bowel sounds.

74. A 60-year-old man post cholecystectomy complains of lower abdominal pain. On examination the bladder is palpable at the umbilicus.

75. A 70-year-old woman post total hip replacement becomes tachypnoeic. She is pale and hypotensive.

Theme: Diagnosis of chest injuries

Options
- A Flail chest
- B Tension pneumothorax
- C Haemothorax
- D Cardiac tamponade
- E Rib fracture
- F Pulmonary contusion
- G Myocardial contusion
- H Diaphragmatic rupture
- I Open pneumothorax

For each case below, choose the SINGLE most likely diagnosis from the above list of options. Each option may be used once, more than once, or not at all.

76. A 50-year-old man sustains blunt trauma to his chest and presents with marked dyspnoea. A nasogastric tube is inserted to decompress his stomach. On chest x-ray the nasogastric tube is seen in the left side of the chest.

77. A 55-year-old man involved in a road traffic accident complains of chest pain. He was driving the car and rear-ended the front car with some force. A friction rub is elicited. ECG shows multiple premature ventricular ectopic beats.

78. A 30-year-old man is stabbed in the back and is brought to Accident and Emergency in respiratory distress. Blood pressure is 90/50 with a pulse rate of 110. There are dull breath sounds over his left chest. You leave the knife in situ.

79. A 40-year-old man is stabbed in the chest and is brought to Accident and Emergency with shortness of breath. A 4-cm stab wound is noted and the wound is heard to 'suck' with each breath.

80. A 30-year-old man is stabbed in the left side of his chest and is brought to Accident and Emergency. He is short of breath and restless. The chest is clear to auscultation. There is a rise in venous pressure with inspiration. Chest x-ray shows a globular shaped heart.

203

Theme: Management of head injuries

Options

A Admit for neurological observation
B Assess adequacy of breathing
C Removal of penetrating object
D Discharge with head injury advice
E Detailed neurological assessment
F Airway assessment with cervical spine control
G Assess circulation and maintain adequate perfusion
H Neurosurgical consultation
I Obtain urgent head CT scan
J Intubate the patient
K Pronounce the patient as deceased

For each case below, choose the SINGLE most appropriate form of management from the above list of options. Each option may be used once, more than once, or not at all.

81. A 30-year-old cyclist is struck by a car in a head-on collision and arrives intubated to Accident and Emergency. Upon arrival his Glasgow Coma Scale is 3. The pupils are fixed and dilated.

82. A 60-year-old man is brought to Accident and Emergency following assault and battery to the head. He has a face mask and reservoir bag delivering 15 L/min of oxygen, a stiff cervical collar and is attached to an intravenous drip. He has no spontaneous eye opening except to pain, makes incomprehensible sounds and does not obey commands. He demonstrates flexion withdrawal to painful stimuli. On suction he has no gag reflex.

83. A 20-year-old man involved in a RTA presents to Accident and Emergency with a large open scalp wound, multiple facial injuries and a deformed right tibia.

84. A 40-year-old man is brought to Casualty with a knife impaled in his occiput.

85. A 30-year-old female involved in a RTA with multiple injuries is brought to Casualty intubated with adequate oxygen delivery. Blood pressure is 80/50 with a pulse of 120.

Theme: Management of back pain

Options

     A Obtain chest x-ray
     B Bedrest for 2 weeks
     C Rest for 2 days with analgaesia
     D Physiotherapy
     E Urinalysis
     F Investigate for underlying tumour or other bone pathology
     G Urgent orthopaedic referral for surgical decompression
     H Routine orthopaedic referral for decompression of nerve root
     I Abdominal ultrasound

For each case below, choose the SINGLE most appropriate management option from the above list of options. Each option may be used once, more than once, or not at all.

86. A 40-year-old man complains of lower back pain after moving heavy furniture. He has no associated nerve root findings.

87. A 50-year-old female complains of back pain worse at night. X-ray of her spine shows crush fractures of two vertebrae. She denies trauma.

88. A 60-year-old man presents with back pain radiating bilaterally below the knees. On examination he has saddle anaesthesia, urinary incontinence and loss of anal tone.

89. A 50-year-old female complains of chronic lower back pain radiating into her buttocks. There is no evidence of nerve root entrapment.

90. A 30-year-old man complains of back pain radiating below the knee. On examination he has sensory loss over the lateral aspect of the right calf and medial aspect of the right foot. He is unable to dorsiflex his great toe. He has tried bedrest for 6 weeks!

Theme: Diagnosis of head injuries

Options

    A Basal skull fracture
    B Depressed skull fracture
    C Compound skull fracture
    D Diffuse axonal injury
    E Concussion
    F Subdural haematoma
    G Intracerebral haemorrhage
    H Extradural haematoma
    I Open skull fracture
    J Brain contusion

For each case below, choose the SINGLE most likely diagnosis from the above list of options. Each option may be used once, more than once, or not at all.

91. A 30-year-old female involved in a RTA is brought by ambulance to Accident and Emergency. There is bruising of the mastoid process and periorbital haematoma. On otoscopic examination there is bleeding behind the tympanic membrane.

92. A 60-year-old man was kicked in the head a week ago. He is brought to Accident and Emergency in an unconscious state. He smells of alcohol. On examination he has a rising BP and unequal pupils. GCS is 8.

93. A 40-year-old man was struck in the head by a cricket ball. He had an episode of loss of consciousness lasting 5 minutes. The patient now complains of headache. He has no lateralising signs on neurological examination.

94. A 50-year-old man with a history of epilepsy has a fit and strikes the side of his head on the edge of the bathtub. He is dazed and complains of headache. Skull x-ray reveals a linear fracture of the parietal area. His level of consciousness diminishes.

95. A 60-year-old man is struck in the head with a dustbin lid and presents with an open scalp wound. Skull x-ray confirms an underlying skull fracture. The dura is intact.

Theme: Treatment of shoulder region injuries

Options

    A Broad arm sling
    B Collar and cuff sling
    C Rest and analgaesia then mobilise
    D Injection of local anaesthetic and steroids
    E Manipulation under anaesthesia
    F Traction on the arm in 90° of abduction and externally rotate
       the arm
    G Hippocratic technique
    H Kocher's technique
    I Surgical repair

For each case below, choose the SINGLE most appropriate treatment from the above list of options. Each option may be used once, more than once, or not at all.

96. A 20-year-old man presents with shoulder pain and decreased range of movement after being struck in the upper back. X-ray reveals fracture of the scapula.

97. A 60-year-old builder presents with pain in the upper arm. On examination there is a low bulge of the muscle belly of the long head of biceps.

98. A 50-year-old man complains of pain in his shoulder. The pain is elicited in abduction between an arc of 60 and 120°. He reports that he has always had shoulder trouble.

99. A 20-year-old rugby player falls onto the point of his shoulder and complains of shoulder tip pain. The lateral end of the clavicle is very prominent.

100. A 30-year-old hiker falls onto his outstretched hand and injures his right shoulder. On examination there is loss of the rounded shoulder contour with prominence of the acromion. On palpation there is a gap beneath the acromion, and the humeral head is palpable in the axilla. The nearest hospital is 6 hours' hike away, and you are alone with him up on the mountain. You cannot obtain a signal on your mobile phone. You decide to treat the patient.

Theme: Causes of a painful foot

Options

    A Morton's neuroma
    B Stress fracture
    C Avulsion fracture
    D Jones fracture
    E Hallux fracture
    F Plantar fasciitis
    G Osteochondritis – Freiberg's disease
    H Metatarsalgia
    I Osteochondritis – Kohler's disease
    J Bunion
    K Gout

For each case below, choose the SINGLE most likely cause from the above list of options. Each option may be used once, more than once, or not at all.

101. A 50-year-old man presents with pain over the medial calcaneum and pain on dorsiflexion and eversion of the forefoot.

102. A 60-year-old man complains of continual pain in his forefoot worse when walking. X-ray shows widening and flattening of the second metatarsal head and degenerative changes in the metatarsophalangeal joint.

103. A 50-year-old woman complains of painful shooting pains in her right foot when walking. There is tenderness in the third/fourth toe interspace.

104. A 30-year-old soldier complains of pain in his foot when weight-bearing. X-ray shows no fracture. There is tenderness around the proximal fifth metatarsal bone.

105. A 20-year-old man complains of pain over the lateral aspect of his right foot. X-ray shows a transverse fracture of the basal shaft of the fifth metatarsal bone.

Theme: Management of ENT emergencies

Options

      A Give nifedipine 10 mg
      B Obtain a barium swallow
      C Obtain a sialogram
      D Advise patient to drink more fluids and avoid citrus fruits
      E List for bronchoscopy
      F List for rigid oesophagoscopy
      G IM buscopan
      H Insert two large-bore intravenous cannulas and run gelofusin
      I Ligate sphenopalatine artery in theatre
      J Consult haematologist
      K Check INR

For each patient below, choose the SINGLE most appropriate management option from the above list of options. Each option may be used once, more than once, or not at all.

106. A 70-year-old woman presents with severe epistaxis. BP is 205/115. She has no prior history of hypertension. She denies aspirin or warfarin use. Bloods are taken, and an intravenous line is inserted. She continues to bleed profusely through her nose packs.

107. A 60-year-old man on warfarin 6 mg od for a previous DVT now presents with right-sided epistaxis. BP is 120/70 with a pulse rate of 90. He has no visible vessels in Little's area. He continues to bleed through the nose pack.

108. A 60-year-old woman presents with a piece of chicken stuck in her throat. Soft-tissue neck x-ray reveals a calcified bolus at the level of the cricopharyngeus.

109. A 70-year-old woman complains of mashed potato stuck in her throat since dinner. She is not distressed. She is able to sip water.

110. A 30-year-old man complains of intermittent unilateral cheek swelling with eating. On examination no swelling is palpated, and the oral cavity is clear.

Theme: Investigations of surgical disease

Options

    A Gastrograffin swallow
    B Upright chest x-ray
    C Abdominal x-ray
    D Full blood count
    E Mesenteric arteriogram
    F CT scan of the abdomen
    G Technetium-99 radioactive scan
    H Abdominal ultrasound
    I Serum urea and electrolytes
    J Stool culture

For each case below, choose the SINGLE most discriminating investigation from the above list of options. Each option may be used once, more than once, or not at all.

111. A 60-year-old man, postop. rigid oesophagoscopy and removal of a foreign body, now presents with substernal pain, fever and tachypnoea.

112. A 65-year-old man with a history of cirrhosis presents with massive rectal bleeding and right lower quadrant pain. NG tube lavage reveals no blood in the stomach. Colonoscopy reveals no varices. You suspect angiodysplasia of the caecum.

113. A 20-year-old man presents with passage of frank blood and clots from his rectum. Blood tests, barium enema and upper GI series are all normal.

114. A 60-year-old man with lung cancer has elevated liver function tests. You suspect metastatic disease.

115. A 65-year-old alcoholic now presents with a tender palpable midline mass. He was recently hospitalised for acute pancreatitis 2 weeks prior. The serum amylase is raised. You now suspect he has a pancreatic pseudocyst.

Theme: Treatment of abdominal pain

Options

     A ERCP and endoscopic sphincterotomy
     B Laparoscopic cholecystectomy
     C IV fluids, IV antibiotics and analgaesia
     D Subtotal colectomy, mucous fistula and permanent ileostomy
     E Laparotomy
     F Mesalazine
     G Panproctocolectomy
     H Hartmann's procedure

For each case below, choose the SINGLE most appropriate treatment from the above list of options. Each option may be used once, more than once, or not at all.

116. A 20-year-old female presents with recurrent bloody diarrhoea and crampy abdominal pain. Sigmoidoscopy and biopsy confirm ulcerative colitis.

117. A 25-year-old man involved in a RTA sustains blunt trauma to his upper abdomen. He complains of left shoulder pain and diffuse abdominal pain. He becomes increasingly tachycardic and hypotensive and develops peritoneal signs.

118. A 40-year-old woman presents with pyrexia and right upper quadrant abdominal pain. The white cell count is 14 with elevated neutrophils. Both the chest x-ray and the abdominal x-ray are unremarkable.

119. A 50-year-old man presents with fever, right upper quadrant pain and jaundice. Ultrasound reveals a dilated common bile duct.

120. A 30-year-old man presents with severe, intractable abdominal pain. He is pyrexial, tachycardic and has marked abdominal distension. On x-ray the colon is noted to have a transverse diameter of 7 cm.

Answers to Surgery SBAs/BOFs

1. A

2. C

3. C

4. E. The patient would be fed via NGT or PEG.

5. A

6. D

7. B

8. B

9. A. Then notify the surgical registrar of your findings.

10. C

11. B

12. B

13. C

14. E

15. B. Oral contraceptives can be a cause of breast pain.

16. A

17. B. Steroids are a risk factor for gastritis.

18. A

19. C

20. A

21. C

22. D

23. E. Two reasons for operating would be cosmetic appearance and compression of the trachea.

24. D. Primary chemotherapy is used to shrink inoperable breast tumours to make them amenable to surgery.

25. B. Follicular thyroid carcinoma implies capsular invasion, which cannot be diagnosed on FNAC. Frozen section is required at hemithyroidectomy.

26. B. Adrenal atrophy is a complication of steroid therapy.

27. C. Ultrasound is used to determine the diameter of the aortic aneurysm. If the diameter is >5.5 cm, there is increased risk of rupture and AAA repair is advocated.

28. B

29. A

30. E

31. C

32. B

33. B

34. B

35. C

36. D. Thiazide diuretics are associated with hypercalcaemia. Loop diuretics are associated with increased calcium excretion.

37. E

38. D. Doppler scan and venous plethysmography will detect 90% of DVTs above the calf veins but miss calf DVTs.

39. E

40. E

41. A. This patient has a bowel ileus and has aspirated probably on a liquid diet into the RLL of the lung.

42. B

43. A

44. B

45. C

46. B

47. D

48. A

49. A

50. C

51. E. Loperamide may precipitate a paralytic ileus and mega-colon.

52. B. A cut over a knuckle is presumed to be a human bite until proven otherwise. Human bite wounds should be left open to heal. Antibiotics are indicated to cover for anaerobic streptococci.

53. C

54. E

55. A

56. C. Tamoxifen is indicated in postmenopausal women with positive oestrogen receptors.

57. E

58. B

59. A

60. C

61. E. Poorer prognosis is associated with BANS (back, back of arms, neck and scalp), trunk and ulcerated malignant melanomas.

62. B

63. E

64. B

65. E. Liver failure results in depleted glycogen stores and consequently results in hypoglycaemia.

66. A. This patient has a pharyngeal pouch. The signs and symptoms are classic and the pouch may be palpable on the left side of the neck.

67. C

68. D. Although gas may be seen in the soft tissues of the neck and around the mediastinum on plain films, a water-based contrast swallow will also localise the perforation. The patient may also have subcutaneous emphysema.

69. C

70. C

71. E

72. D. The neck of a femoral hernia is narrow and more likely to incarcerate.

73. B

74. C

75. A

76. B

77. E

78. C. TURP syndrome may occur if the operation is prolonged, i.e. >1 hour, and excessive fluid irrigation is used.

79. E

80. C

81. E. PET is not readily available.

82. D

83. B

84. A. Percutaneous nephrostomy is advised initially to relieve renal obstruction.

85. B. Cefuroxime is the antibiotic of choice for clean surgery with prosthetic material.

86. C. Metronidazole PR is advised 4 hours preop. appendicectomy.

87. E

88. D. 1–2 doses of vancomycin are indicated to cover against *Staphylococcus aureus* and coagulase-negative staphylococci.

89. E

90. E

91. C

92. D. Antimuscarinic agents are used in the treatment of urinary frequency.

93. C

94. B

95. E

96. D

97. B. Erosion of the anterior wall and into the innominate artery can result in catastrophic bleeding and death.

98. D

99. A

100. E

101. E

102. E. The patient should be treated for hypercalcaemic crisis secondary to malignancy.

103. D. Signs of venous hypertension should be checked, not arterial insufficiency.

104. D

105. A

106. B. Gas gangrene is one of the indications for BKA.

107. C

108. A

109. C

110. E

111. B

112. D

113. E

114. B

115. B

116. A. The patient is shocked and not stable enough for a CT scan. Take the patient directly to theatre.

117. E

118. E

119. E

120. D

121. A

122. E. Ultrasound is useful to exclude effusion in the hip or septic arthritis.

123. C. Daily temperature checks are necessary to rule out septic arthritis.

124. B

125. A

126. B

127. A. This is physiological fluid for an infant and is used to pull back hydrogen ions from the kidney and excrete potassium. It is the treatment for hypochloraemic alkalosis.

128. B

129. C. This condition is often misdiagnosed as epididymo-orchitis, so beware!

130. D

131. B. This man has angiodysplasia, which is usually localised to the right colon.

132. D

133. C. This lady has acute diverticulitis with peritoneal signs and requires urgent laparotomy.

134. A. Duke's stage A is associated with a 92% 5-year survival rate, Duke's stage C1 with a 40% rate, C2 with a 26.5% rate and D with a 16.4% survival rate at 5 years.

135. D. Dupuytren's contracture is associated with liver disease.

136. E

137. A. This man has stigmata of alcohol liver disease and portal hypertension.

138. E

139. A

140. B

141. C

142. C. 'Pus somewhere, pus nowhere, pus under the diaphragm.' Be alert when confronted with a patient with a persistent swinging pyrexia of unknown origin, occurring several days postop. There is usually a hidden abscess or, in this case, a subphrenic abscess.

143. A. This man most likely requires blood replacement as a lengthy operation is often associated with greater blood loss.

144. C. Blood group A and not O is associated with stomach cancer. Sister Mary Joseph's sign is the association of a hard umbilical nodule with poorer prognosis for intra-abdominal malignancy (i.e. sign of gastric carcinoma metastasis). She was Dr William Mayo's surgical assistant.

145. B

146. E

147. E

148. A

149. E. Blood group A is associated with stomach cancer and not oesophageal cancer.

150. E

151. D. The first two ribs are the hardest to break.

152. D

153. B. This patient needs urgent referral to a specialist hospital centre as cardiopulmonary bypass is required for thoracic aortic arch repair. Leave the specialist centre to organise the CT scan. If it is normal, the centre can send back the patient to you. You will not have lost any time.

154. E

155. B

156. E. Radical gastrectomy is offered for stages I–III.

157. B. This patient should receive palliative care.

158. B

159. C. IV opiates should be administered for analgaesia.

160. C

161. E

162. D

163. C

164. A. BNF guidelines state that 7 days of triple therapy is adequate to eradicate 90% of cases of *H. pylori*. Any longer and patient compliance is poor due to the side-effects of the medications.

165. E

166. E

167. C

168. E

169. C

170. C

171. A

172. A

173. E

174. A. This patient has a positive Pemberton's sign. Raising her arms above her head decreases the size of the thoracic inlet and worsens symptoms.

175. A. The sternum can also be percussed.

176. B

177. D

178. A

179. A

180. E

Answers to Surgery EMQs

1. A. Classic presentation for acute appendicitis.

2. G. Gallstones and alcohol are the main predisposing factors for acute pancreatitis.

3. H. Chronic active hepatitis is associated with methyldopa and also isoniazid.

4. B. Chronic diverticular disease mimics colon cancer but as the latter is not a listed option, chronic diverticular disease is the obvious diagnosis.

5. J

6. F. Axillary lymphadenopathy is indicative of malignancy.

7. B

8. E

9. J. Paget's disease or intraductal carcinoma is associated with eczema of the nipple especially in the presence of a firm nodule suggestive of more than simple eczema.

10. H

11. I

12. D. A thyroglossal cyst moves on swallowing or protrusion of the tongue. The fact that the swelling transilluminates excludes a thyroid swelling.

13. F

14. A

15. B. Ludwig's angina, a submandibular abscess, usually arises from an abscess of the lower premolars or the first and second molar.

16. D

m/

17. I

18. G

19. H

20. C

21. B. Chvostek's sign is demonstrated here and is associated with hypocalcaemia.

22. A. Upright chest x-ray to look for free air under the diaphragm to exclude perforated peptic ulcer disease is suggested here.

23. J. Blood loss from a hip fracture often warrants blood replacement.

24. H. Pulmonary embolism is suggested here.

25. I. Epidural anaesthesia may be associated with urinary retention.

26. H. The presentation is suggestive of ureteric colic.

27. I. The presentation is suggestive of ovarian cyst.

28. C. The presentation is suggestive of peptic ulcer disease.

29. A. The presentation is suggestive of abdominal aortic aneurysm. The size should be evaluated by ultrasound and surgical repair is advisable if the aneurysm is greater than 5 cm in diameter.

30. K. Steroid usage for rheumatoid arthritis puts this lady at risk for a perforated peptic ulcer.

31. A. Presbyacusis is confirmed by pure tone audiogram which would demonstrate symmetrical high-frequency sensorineural hearing loss.

32. D. Syringing, cotton bud usage and swimming are recognised risk factors for otitis externa.

33. I. A conductive hearing loss with a normal tympanic membrane is suggestive of otosclerosis.

34. E. Chronic secretory otitis media or glue ear is treated with watchful waiting for 3 months. If spontaneous resolution has not occurred, referral to an ENT specialist may be necessary.

35. H. This patient has a false-negative Rinne test suggestive of dead ear.

36. H

37. K

38. C

39. A

40. E

41. D

42. K

43. C

44. E

45. F

46. I. Courvoisier's law states that, 'if in a case of painless jaundice, the gallbladder is palpable, the cause will not be gallstones'.

47. K

48. A. Acute appendicitis is less likely without nausea and Crohn's ileitis is less likely without diarrhoea.

49. G. Carcinoma of the caecum is associated with bleeding.

50. E. The commonest presentation of carcinoma of the sigmoid is changes in bowel habit rather than pain.

51. C. Beck's triad consists of muffled heart sounds, hypotension and Kussmaul's sign and is pathognomonic for cardiac tamponade.

52. G

53. M. Absence of the psoas shadow is due to retroperitoneal fluid.

54. I

55. K. Addisonian crisis is precipitated here by omission of doses of a longterm steroid regime.

56. B. In a fit man under 60, AO cannulated screws are preferable to an Austin Moore hemiarthroplasty.

57. F. Anterior cruciate ligament injury should be repaired surgically especially in a young athlete.

58. I. Dynamic hip screw is the standard treatment for intertrochanteric fractures.

59. D. Scapholunate disassociation is repaired by open reduction of the subluxation and a K wire to hold the reduction. The wrist is then splinted.

60. K. Anterior shoulder fracture-dislocation requires open reduction and fixation.

61. I. Dysphagia, stridor, dysphonia or an expanding neck haematoma are all indications to explore a penetrating neck wound.

62. H

63. C. Prompt insertion of a needle or chest tube into the left pleural space is indicated to relieve the pneumothorax.

64. I. Immediate surgical exploration is warranted. An on-table angiogram can be obtained simultaneously.

65. I. Traumatic diaphragmatic rupture is associated with deceleration injuries and requires prompt surgical exploration.

66. J

67. K. Divarication of the rectus abdominis muscles is associated with multiple pregnancies and chronic abdominal distension. The gap is palpable on examination.

68. I. Spontaneous splenic rupture following minor blunt trauma is associated with infectious mononucleosis.

69. B. Bleeding oesophageal varices are often the cause of massive haematemesis in children.

70. B

71. A. Malignant hyperthermia may be precipitated by halothane or by succinylcholine.

72. B. Chvostek's sign is a sign of hypocalcaemia, which may occur following thyroidectomy and injury to the parathyroid glands.

73. E. Aspiration pneumonia may occur in a patient with postoperative ileus, drowsiness or with altered swallowing.

74. I. This patient is in urinary retention.

75. K. This patient may need blood replacement.

76. H. Diaphragmatic rupture can be diagnosed on chest x-ray by the presence of bowel or the nasogastric tube being seen in the chest.

77. G. This usually arises from chest injury sustained by hitting the steering wheel with great force.

78. C

79. I. Open pneumothorax is treated by covering the wound with a piece of gauze which is taped down along three sides to act as a flutter-valve.

80. D. Kussmaul's sign is a classic sign for cardiac tamponade as is Beck's triad. However not all patients present with classic signs!

81. K. A Glasgow Coma Scale (GCS) of 3 is the lowest score possible.

82. J. A GCS of 8 or less or absence of a gag reflex are both indications for intubation.

83. F. No mention of airway management has been made and therefore should be included in the initial assessment of this patient.

84. F. Penetrating objects should be left in situ until surgery. Again airway assessment is always the first priority in management of head injuries.

85. G. Hypotension should not be assumed to be caused by brain injury.

86. C. Acute back strain is treated conservatively.

87. F. Night pain and pathological fractures should make one suspicious for underlying pathology.

88. G. Acute cauda equina syndrome requires urgent decompression.

89. D. Mechanical back pain is treated conservatively.

90. H. Intervertebral disc prolapse is the commonest cause of root pain.

91. A. Battle's sign (bruising over the mastoid process), raccoon eyes (periorbital bruising), haemotympanum and CSF leak in the ears or nose are all signs associated with basal skull fracture.

92. F

93. E. Concussion is the transient loss of consciousness without accompanying neurological signs.

94. H

95. C. If the dura was breached, the diagnosis is one of open skull fracture.

96. A

97. C. Surgical repair is undertaken in athletes or associated rotator cuff tear injuries.

98. D. Painful arc syndrome is treated with injections of local anaesthetic and steroids. The syndrome is due to degenerative changes of the supraspinatus tendon.

99. A. Acromioclavicular joint subluxation or dislocation is treated conservatively with a broad arm sling followed by mobilisation.

100. G. The Hippocratic technique is a one-man technique as opposed to Kocher's manoeuvre which requires an assistant for counter-traction. Pain may be a limiting factor to successful reduction.

101. F

102. G

103. A

104. B. A bone scan may be necessary to confirm a stress fracture.

105. D

106. A. Hypertension will contribute to ongoing epistaxis. Nifedipine is advisable to lower the patient's BP. She will then need to see her GP for regular antihypertensive therapy.

107. K. Any patient on warfarin who presents with epistaxis should have a clotting screen checked. Treatment with vitamin K may be required. However, the haematologist should be consulted for advice if this is the case.

108. F. A food bolus containing bone is at high risk for perforating the oesophagus and needs prompt attention.

109. G. This patient can be managed conservatively at first with buscopan, a muscle antispasmodic. She will need an outpatient barium swallow upon discharge.

110. D. This patient will need a sialogram if the parotid swelling reoccurs.

111. A. A chest x-ray may show air in the soft tissues but a gastrograffin swallow is conclusive in the diagnosis of oesophageal perforation.

112. E

113. G. A technetium scan should be arranged to investigate for Meckel's diverticula.

114. F

115. H

116. F. Medical therapy should be initiated. Mesalazine is a newer aminosalicylate that avoids the side-effects of sulfasalazine.

117. E. The liver and spleen are at high risk of injury from blunt trauma to the abdomen.

118. C. Acute cholecystitis is managed conservatively until an urgent ultrasound can be arranged.

119. A

120. D. This patient has toxic megacolon and is at high risk of perforation when the transverse diameter of the colon exceeds 6 cm.

In these questions candidates must select one answer only

Questions

1. A 70-year-old woman requests to be started on an anti-depressant for a 1-year history of depression. She has a history of poorly controlled epilepsy. Which medication would you commence?

   A. donepezil
   B. dothiepin
   C. MAOI
   D. sertraline (SSRI)
   E. venlafaxine

2. A 40-year-old man is diagnosed with schizophrenia. What is the most appropriate first-line outpatient medication?

   A. clozapine
   B. haloperidol
   C. chlorpromazine
   D. olanzapine
   E. piportal

3. Which blood test should be arranged for this patient on this medication?

   A. FBC and LFTs
   B. FBC and INR
   C. urea/electrolytes and calcium
   D. FBC and urea/electrolytes
   E. FBC, glucose and calcium

4. The following drugs are recognised treatment for bipolar disorder EXCEPT:

A. sodium valproate
B. lithium
C. carbamazepine
D. SSRIs
E. phenytoin

5. A 55-year-old homeless man is brought to Casualty. The police are concerned for his welfare. On examination, he is unkempt with dirty fingernails and talks very quietly. He hesitates briefly before he responds appropriately to your questions. His face does not change expression. The most likely diagnosis is:

A. depression
B. schizophrenia
C. Parkinson's disease
D. hypothyroidism
E. temporal lobe epilepsy

6. Appropriate initial investigations for this man include all of the following EXCEPT:

A. FBC
B. TFTs
C. urine toxicology
D. calcium and glucose
E. electroencephalogram

7. Immediate side-effects of antipsychotic drugs include all of the following EXCEPT:

A. tardive dyskinesia
B. dystonias
C. oculogyric crisis
D. neuroleptic malignant syndrome
E. akathisia

8. Which of the following evidence-based questionnaires is used for postnatal depression?

    A. Hamilton
    B. Beck
    C. Edinburgh
    D. MAST
    E. CAGE

9. A 40-year-old inpatient being treated for paranoid schizophrenia threatens to leave the hospital. Under which Section of the Mental Health Act of 1983 can he be detained by you as a house officer?

    A. 2
    B. 3
    C. 4
    D. 5
    E. 7

10. A 30-year-old woman is brought to Casualty by the police under Section 136 of the Mental Health Act of 1983 for self-neglect. Under which Section can she then be admitted and detained for 72 hours?

    A. 2
    B. 3
    C. 4
    D. 5
    E. 12

11. A 40-year-old woman has been grieving for 18 months for her deceased child. She is both depressed and anxious all the time. Appropriate management includes all of the following EXCEPT:

    A. SSRIs
    B. benzodiazepines
    C. cognitive behaviour therapy
    D. buspirone
    E. EMDR (eye movement desensitisation and reprocessing)

12. A 20-year-old woman complains of recurrent episodes of chest pains, hot flushes, paraesthesias and difficulty breathing. The episodes peak in severity within 10 minutes. After exclusion of any physical aetiology, appropriate management includes all of the following EXCEPT:

A. fast-acting benzodiazepine
B. tricyclic antidepressant
C. cognitive-behaviour therapy
D. SSRI
E. MAOI

13. A 20-year-old woman presents with chest pain. She is wearing baggy trousers and an oversized jumper. You suspect anorexia nervosa. Her height is 1.5 m and her weight is 36 kg. What is her body mass index (BMI)?

A. 15
B. 16
C. 17
D. 20
E. 24

14. A 55-year-old woman complains of depression for 6 months. She has lost interest in sex, food and suffers insomnia. Appropriate investigations include all of the following EXCEPT:

A. prolactin
B. FBC
C. glucose
D. TFTs
E. LFTs

15. The FSH/LH level comes back as 20 IU/L. What is the most appropriate treatment to offer?

A. HRT
B. SSRI
C. benzodiazepine
D. psychosexual counselling
E. refer to gynaecologist

16. A 55-year-old man who suffers from alcoholism is hospitalised for acute alcoholic hepatitis. The liver unit would like you to commence alcohol detoxification. The most appropriate drug to use is:

    A. heminevrin (chlormethiazole)
    B. diazepam
    C. acamprosate
    D. disulfiram
    E. lofexidine

17. A 20-year-old IV drug abuser requests drug therapy. He injects 1.5 g of heroin daily and uses 2 rocks a week. What is the first step in management?

    A. take urine for toxicology to confirm presence of opiates
    B. take blood for FBC and LFTs
    C. take blood for hepatitis B, C and HIV test
    D. commence methadone at 20 ml daily on a daily pick-up basis
    E. commence buprenorphine therapy at an initial dose of 4 mg

18. A 25-year-old man is brought to Casualty obtunded. He has no physical signs of head trauma. He has needle marks on his neck and groin. His pupils are pinpoint. His respiratory rate is 6 per minute. He is receiving 100% oxygen by face mask. The next most immediate management would be:

    A. urine for toxicology
    B. naloxone IV injection
    C. endotracheal intubation
    D. flumazenil antidote
    E. arterial blood gas

19. A 55-year old man admitted for alcohol detoxification suddenly starts fitting in front of you on the ward. What is the initial treatment for status epilepticus?

    A. rectal diazepam
    B. intramuscular diazepam
    C. intravenous diazepam
    D. intravenous phenytoin sodium
    E. rectal paraldehyde

20. A 40-year-old man who was a passenger in a serious RTA complains of flashbacks, hypervigiliance, insomnia and poor concentration. Recognised treatment includes all of the following EXCEPT:

A. benzodiazepines
B. antidepressants
C. beta-blockers
D. assertiveness training
E. debriefing

21. High-risk indicators for suicide include all of the following EXCEPT:

A. male
B. family history of suicide
C. drug abuse
D. depression
E. age <40 years

22. Schneider's symptoms of the first rank suggestive of the diagnosis of schizophrenia include all of the following EXCEPT:

A. delusional perception
B. somatic passivity
C. flat affect
D. thought block
E. third person auditory hallucinations

23. A 23-year-old woman presents with a history of catastrophic mood swings, intense and multiple relationships, and describes her life as emotional chaos. She has cut herself in the past to relieve emotional pain. She drinks alcohol and indulges in cannabis. Her family states that she has always been like this and likens her to a 2-year-old having a tantrum. The most likely diagnosis is:

A. bipolar disorder
B. borderline personality disorder
C. schizotypal disorder
D. antisocial personality disorder
E. histrionic personality disorder

24. A 40-year-old patient has been on fluoxetine for 3 months and asks when he should discontinue the medication, as he is feeling much better now. You advise him to continue for:

A. I month
B. 6 weeks
C. 3 months
D. 6 months
E. I year

25. Side-effects of tricyclic antidepressants include all of the following EXCEPT:

A. postural hypotension
B. drowsiness
C. agranulocytosis
D. convulsions
E. cardiotoxicity

26. A 70-year-old woman on dothiepin, a tricyclic antidepressant, presents with convulsions. The most useful blood test is:

A. FBC
B. INR
C. LFTs
D. sodium
E. potassium

27. A 40-year-old woman complains that she has had no response to fluoxetine 20 mg od for her depression after 8 weeks. She also complains of chronic anxiety and insomnia. The next line of drug for depression would be:

A. venlafaxine
B. MAOI
C. benzodiazepine
D. tricyclic antidepressant
E. moclobemide

28. Appropriate measures in dealing with aggressive patients include all of the following EXCEPT:

A. lower the pitch of your voice
B. keep your hands in full view of the patient
C. be punctual
D. sit facing the patient
E. position yourself closer to the door

29. Physical disorders that may mimic anxiety include all of the following EXCEPT:

A. carcinoid syndrome
B. alcohol intoxication
C. excessive caffeine
D. thyrotoxicosis
E. hypoglycaemia

30. A 40-year-old woman complains of several months of anxiety, insomnia, irritability and depression following an acrimonious divorce. She requests medication to help her sleep. Appropriate treatment may include all of the following EXCEPT:

A. short-term benzodiazepine
B. referral for counselling
C. buspirone
D. SSRI
E. beta-blocker

31. A 50-year-old man reports consuming the equivalent of 36 units of alcohol a week. The most appropriate screening test for problem drinking is:

A. CAGE
B. gamma-glutamyl transferase
C. mean corpuscular volume
D. the presence of spider naevi
E. the presence of a tender liver edge

32. A 45-year-old man reports a daily alcohol consumption of 2 cans of extra strong lager. He complains of hearing rustling sounds and disturbing voices while drinking. What is the most appropriate management?

    A. admit the patient immediately to hospital
    B. commence an atypical antipsychotic medication, i.e. olanzapine
    C. commence a typical psychotic medication, i.e. haloperidol
    D. commence chlormethiazole
    E. commence diazepam

33. Alcohol consumption is associated with all of the following EXCEPT:

    A. 80% of suicides
    B. half of all hospital admissions
    C. 40% of RTAs
    D. 80% of deaths from fire
    E. I in 3 cases of child abuse

34. A 40-year-old man with longstanding schizophrenia now presents with fever and impaired consciousness. On examination there is muscle rigidity, a labile blood pressure and tachycardia. Serum creatinine kinase is raised. The most likely diagnosis is:

    A. septicaemia
    B. tardive dyskinesia
    C. neuroleptic malignant syndrome
    D. acute myocardial infarction
    E. meningitis

35. A 55-year-old man is taking lithium for bipolar disorder. In addition to checking the blood levels of lithium, the following tests should be arranged every 3 months EXCEPT for:

    A. LFTs
    B. TFTs
    C. FBC
    D. ECG
    E. urea/electrolytes

36. A 20-year-old woman states that she is usually up all night doing one thing or another. She describes herself as a very busy woman with lots of new and exciting projects. She gets annoyed with her family for being obstructive to some of her plans. She admits to shopping excessively. Her family reports that she has always been a busy-bee. What is the most likely diagnosis?

A. borderline personality disorder (emotionally unstable)
B. anankastic (obsessional) personality
C. bipolar disorder
D. obsessive-compulsive disorder
E. drug or alcohol addiction

37. Causes of erectile dysfunction include all of the following EXCEPT:

A. diabetes mellitus
B. SSRI therapy
C. methadone therapy
D. alcohol
E. hypertension

38. Features of heroin withdrawal syndrome include all of the following EXCEPT:

A. insomnia
B. muscle cramps
C. diarrhoea
D. yawning
E. pinpoint pupils

39. Complications produced by IV drug abuse include all of the following EXCEPT:

A. hepatitis C
B. deep vein thrombosis
C. hepatitis A
D. thrombophlebitis
E. cellulitis

40. Features of benzodiazepine withdrawal syndrome include all of the following EXCEPT:

    A. anxiety
    B. hallucinations
    C. tinnitus
    D. heightened sensitivity to light
    E. pinpoint pupils

41. Drug treatments for Alzheimer's disease include all of the following EXCEPT:

    A. donepezil
    B. lovasatatin
    C. galantamine
    D. rivastigmine
    E. selegiline

42. Characteristic features of dementia include all of the following EXCEPT:

    A. abrupt onset
    B. aggressive outbursts
    C. decrement in memory and judgment
    D. poor social and personal relationships
    E. clear consciousness

43. Reversible causes of dementia include all of the following EXCEPT:

    A. hypothyroidism
    B. hypoparathyroidism
    C. communicating hydrocephalus
    D. vitamin B_{12} deficiency
    E. renal failure

44. Negative symptoms of schizophrenia include all of the following EXCEPT:

    A. poverty of thought
    B. blunted affect
    C. auditory hallucinations
    D. social withdrawal
    E. poverty of speech

45. Potential side-effects of atypical antipsychotics include all of the following EXCEPT:

    A. weight loss
    B. agranulocytosis
    C. hepatitis
    D. extrapyramidal symptoms
    E. postural hypotension

46. Features of schizophrenia include all of the following EXCEPT:

    A. ambivalence
    B. loosening of associations
    C. autism
    D. loss of affect
    E. excessive anxiety

47. You are called to the ward to see a 45-year-old acutely disturbed patient. He cannot be calmed. You decide he requires rapid tranquillisation. He has no history of heart disease. The nurses restrain the patient while you inject which medication?

    A. droperidol 10 mg IM + lorazepam 2 mg IM
    B. depot antipsychotic (piportil) IM
    C. zuclopenthixol acetate 100–150 mg IM
    D. chlorpromazine 25 mg IM
    E. morphine 10 mg IV

48. Components of the mental state examination include all of the following EXCEPT:

    A. speech
    B. appearance
    C. diagnosis
    D. perception
    E. intellect

49. Side-effects of tricyclic antidepressants include all of the following EXCEPT:

    A. bradycardia
    B. weight gain
    C. dry mouth
    D. disturbance of eye accommodation
    E. increased intraocular pressure

50. A 60-year-old man with schizophrenia requires compulsory admission to hospital for treatment of his disorder. Under which Section of the Mental Health Act of 1983 should he be admitted for treatment?

    A. 2
    B. 3
    C. 4
    D. 5
    E. 7

51. Features of childhood autism include all of the following EXCEPT:

    A. abnormal response to pain
    B. imitation
    C. echolalia
    D. avoids mutual gaze
    E. impaired imagination

52. Features of delirium include all of the following EXCEPT:

    A. clouding of consciousness
    B. gradual, stepwise onset
    C. perseveration
    D. delusions
    E. labile mood

53. Strategies in long-term psychotherapy include all of the following EXCEPT:

    A. reflecting
    B. linking
    C. free association
    D. confrontation
    E. paternalism

54. Indications for electroconvulsive therapy may include all of the following EXCEPT:

    A. high suicide risk
    B. psychotic depression
    C. depression unresponsive to antidepressants
    D. post-traumatic stress disorder
    E. depression with marked psychomotor retardation

55. Medical presentations of alcoholism include all of the following EXCEPT:

    A. memory loss
    B. gastritis
    C. pancreatitis
    D. hypertension
    E. carcinoma of the prostate

56. Complications of delirium tremens include all of the following EXCEPT:

    A. hypothermia
    B. dehydration
    C. convulsions
    D. chest infection
    E. electrolyte imbalance

57. Organic causes of mania include all of the following EXCEPT:

    A. HIV infection
    B. malaria
    C. hypothyroidism
    D. cerebral tumour
    E. SLE

58. Medium duration (weeks) side-effects of antipsychotic drugs include all of the following EXCEPT:

    A. amenorrhoea
    B. impotence
    C. prolonged QTc interval
    D. weight gain
    E. tardive dyskinesias

59. Features of mania may include all of the following EXCEPT:

    A. flight of ideas
    B. pressure of speech
    C. irritability
    D. evident in early life
    E. grandiose beliefs

60. The following statements are true EXCEPT for:

A. Paroxetine is the most sedating SSRI.
B. MAOIs may be safely initiated in a primary care setting.
C. Clozapine may require inpatient administration.
D. If a patient on haloperidol 10 mg od is experiencing parkinsonian side-effects, the dose is sufficient to block dopamine receptors in the limbic system.
E. Memory loss has been reported following ECT.

Psychiatry EMQS
Theme: Treatment of psychiatric conditions

Options

A Buprenorphine (subutex)
B Clozapine
C Amitryptiline
D Diazepam
E Carbamazepine
F Olanzapine (atypical antipsychotic)
G SSRI
H Lofexidine
I Heminevrin
J Electroconvulsive therapy
K Haloperidol
L Sodium valproate
M Lithium
N Venlafaxine
O Acamprosate

For each patient below, choose the SINGLE most likely diagnosis from the above list of options. Each option may be used once, more than once, or not at all.

1. A 30-year-old IV drug abuser asks for heroin detoxification therapy. He has tried a methadone regime of 30 ml od without success and would like to try something new. His urine screen confirms the presence of heroin, methadone and cocaine.

2. A 50-year-old alcoholic requests alcohol detoxification therapy. You refer him to a local community inpatient detox centre. Which drug will he be given?

3. A 20-year-old woman complains of depression lasting for 1 year. You evaluate her depression as moderate. Which drug would you commence?

4. A 30-year-old man presents with obtrusive auditory hallucinations that tell him to kill himself. He informs you that he will not harm himself. Which medication would you consider commencing?

5. A 55-year-old man requests medication to help him resist alcohol. He has completed an alcohol detox programme. Which drug would you commence?

Theme: Diagnosis of psychiatric disorders

Options

A   Suicidal risk
B   Alcohol abuse
C   Generalised anxiety
D   Dementia
E   Panic attacks
F   Bipolar disorder
G   Drug abuse
H   Depression
I   Delirium
J   Grief reaction
K   Schizophrenia
L   Borderline personality disorder

For each patient below, choose the SINGLE most likely diagnosis from the above list of options. Each option may be used once, more than once, or not at all.

6. A 70-year-old retired engineer experiences changes in personality and impaired social skills. This is corroborated by his family, who describe him as forgetful and not as sharp.

7. A 20-year-old man is noted to be withdrawn, isolated and 'peculiar'. He experiences persecutory delusions and auditory hallucinations. His urine toxicology screen is clear.

8. A 60-year-old widow is noted by her family to be restless, disorganised, crying, and frequently expresses her wish to join her deceased partner.

9. A 40-year-old Irishman complains of frequent episodes of chest pains, sweating, palpitations, a sense of impending doom and paraesthesias that last for minutes at a time.

10. A 25-year-old man presents with miosis, slurred speech, disorientation and respiratory depression.

Theme: Treatment of psychiatric disorders

Options

- A Long-term psychotherapy
- B Lithium
- C Donepezil, a reverse inhibitor of acetylcholinesterase
- D Levodopa in combination with a dopa-decarboxylase inhibitor
- E Diazepam
- F Haloperidol
- G Tetrabenazine
- H Propranolol
- I Disulfiram
- J Methadone
- K Fluoxetine

For each case below, choose the SINGLE most appropriate treatment from the above list of options. Each option may be used once, more than once, or not at all.

11. A 70-year-old man presents with progressive forgetfulness and mood changes. He has a shuffling gait. CT scan of the head shows cortical atrophy and enlarged ventricles.

12. A 60-year-old man presents with a disturbance of voluntary motor function. His face is expressionless. On examination cogwheel rigidity and bradykinesia are present.

13. A 10-year-old boy presents with brief, repetitive motor tics and is brought in by his parents for shouting obscenities at school.

14. A 40-year-old man presents with ataxia. His wife states that it runs in her husband's family. He is difficult to live with, very irritable, clumsy and suffers from jerky movements of the legs.

15. A 20-year-old man presents with sweating, muscle twitching and abdominal cramps. On examination the pupils are dilated.

Theme: Diagnosis of organic mental disorders

Options

- A Parkinson's disease
- B Huntington's disease
- C Alzheimer's disease
- D Multi-infarct dementia
- E Creutzfeldt–Jakob disease
- F Korsakoff's psychosis
- G Temporal lobe seizures
- H Wernicke's encephalopathy
- I Chronic subdural haematoma
- J Subarachnoid haemorrhage
- K Acute intermittent porphyria

For each patient below, choose the SINGLE most likely diagnosis from the above list of options. Each option may be used once, more than once, or not at all.

16. A 70-year-old man presents with gradual deterioration of memory and intellect. His family has noticed a change in personality and behaviour.

17. A 35-year-old man presents with dementia and choreiform movements.

18. A 60-year-old man with alcohol dependence presents with deterioration of both retrograde and anterograde memory. He invents stories.

19. A 60-year-old man with alcohol dependence presents with persistent headache. His family notes that he is inattentive and becoming more confused.

20. A 65-year-old man presents with an abrupt onset of confusion and ataxia. On examination, nystagmus is present. He is a known drinker.

Theme: Diagnosis of psychiatric disorders

Options

A Schizophrenia
B Brief reactive psychosis
C Bipolar disorder
D Major depression
E Body dysmorphic disorder
F Panic disorder
G Post-traumatic stress disorder
H Schizoaffective disorder
I Delusional disorder
J Paranoid schizophrenia
K Postpartum depression
L Dysthymia

For each patient below, choose the SINGLE most likely diagnosis from the above list of options. Each option may be used once, more than once or not at all.

21. A 40-year-old man insists that his wife is unfaithful and sleeping with the entire neighbourhood. He is hypersensitive, argumentative and litiginous. His wife has left him due to his behaviour. He functions well at work.

22. A 25-year-old woman presents with personality changes. She is noted by friends initially to be anxious, irritable and an insomniac and weeks later she becomes profoundly depressed with low self-esteem and contemplates suicide. In consultation she has pressured speech with boundless energy.

23. A 20-year-old woman has a 'mental breakdown'. She has recently broken up with her boyfriend. She has dramatic mood swings, memory loss and incoherent speech. This lasts for a month.

24. A 20-year-old woman presents to her GP complaining of feeling depressed ever since she can remember. Her parents died in a car crash 10 years ago. She sees herself as a failure, but functions well at work. She has trouble falling asleep.

25. A 50-year-old woman complains of sudden episodes of feeling impending doom. During these episodes she feels choked and sweats profusely.

Theme: Diagnosis of psychiatric conditions

Options

     A Pica
     B Formication
     C Alcohol withdrawal
     D Alcohol intoxication
     E Schizophrenia
     F Xenophobia
     G Agoraphobia
     H Algophobia
     I Delirium
     J Fugue
     K Cocaine intoxication
     L Opioid withdrawal
     M Drug toxicity

For each patient below, choose the SINGLE most likely diagnosis from the above list of options. Each option may be used once, more than once, or not at all.

26. A 2-year-old boy presents with anaemia and abdominal pain. His mother states that she has seen him peeling paint chips off the wall and wonders if he has been eating this.

27. A 23-year-old woman becomes afraid to leave her home. She functions normally except will not step outside her house.

28. An 18-year-old man presents with nausea, vomiting and diaphoresis. He has dilated pupils. Blood pressure is elevated. He has a history of drug addiction.

29. A 30-year-old woman is found in an amnestic state. Her husband reports that she had been missing for a few days after she had been served with divorce papers.

30. A 30-year-old man takes lithium for longstanding bipolar disorder. He was recently started on thiazide diuretics for mild hypertension and is now confused with ataxia, blurred vision and a coarse tremor.

Theme: Diagnosis of psychiatric disorders

Options

    A Munchausen's syndrome
    B Alcohol withdrawal delirium
    C Extrapyramidal side-effect
    D Hypothyroidism
    E Hysterical neurosis
    F Acromegaly
    G Dissociative disorder
    H Malingering disorder
    I Parkinson's disease
    J Cushing's syndrome
    K Autonomic side-effect of drug
    L Anticholinergic side-effect of drug

For each patient below, choose the SINGLE most likely diagnosis from the above list of options. Each option may be used once, more than once, or not at all.

31. A 28-year-old female presents with lower abdominal pain. On examination there are multiple surgical scars over her abdomen. Abdominal and pelvic examinations are normal. She insists she needs a laparoscopy.

32. A 50-year-old man with schizophrenia is started on haloperidol. A month later he is noted to be drooling saliva and walking with a shuffling gait. He also suffers from involuntary chewing movements.

33. A 40-year-old female complains of dry mouth, blurry vision and constipation. On examination she has dilated pupils. She was started on amitryptiline for major depression.

34. A 45-year-old man complains of headaches, excessive thirst and frequent urination. On examination he is noted to have bad acne, coarse skin and has a goitre. He has moved his wedding band to the 5th finger.

35. A 30-year-old man presents to Casualty with a dislocated shoulder. On examination the shoulder is found not to be dislocated. The patient insists it is dislocated, and he needs morphine for the pain.

Theme: Diagnosis of conditions that mimic physical disease

Options

A Conversion disorder
B Histrionic personality disorder
C Body dysmorphic disorder
D Briquet's syndrome
E Munchausen's syndrome
F Hypochondriacal neurosis
G Somatoform pain disorder

For each patient below, choose the SINGLE most likely diagnosis from the above list of options. Each option may be used once, more than once, or not at all.

36. A 40-year-old man insists that his leg is gangrenous and needs to be amputated. On examination, he has normal extremities.

37. A 30-year-old woman presents with a history of multi-organ ailments. She reports that she has always been poorly ever since she was a child. She sees her GP on a regular basis and each time for a different medical symptom. No medical abnormalities can be found. She has multiple surgical scars over her entire body.

38. A 50-year-old man facing redundancy is now paralysed in both legs and wheel-chair bound. The paralysis and sensory loss is inconsistent with the anatomical distribution of nerves.

39. A 40-year-old woman after failing her driving test complains of chest pain. No medical cause can be identified.

40. A 50-year-old man insists he has throat cancer. He has 'shopped around' and can find no doctor who will concur with him.

Answers to Psychiatry SBAs/BOFs

1. D

2. D. Newer atypical antipsychotics are now recognised first-line therapy for schizophrenia over typical antipsychotic agents such as haloperidol.

3. A

4. E. Sodium valproate is first-line treatment for bipolar disorder.

5. B

6. E

7. A

8. C

9. D

10. C

11. E. EMDR is a recognised treatment for post-traumatic stress disorder and helps alleviate flashbacks.

12. E

13. B. Body mass index = wt (kg)/ht (metres)^2.

14. A

15. A. An FSH/LH ratio >15 IU/L confirms menopause.

16. B. Heminevrin is no longer recommended as attenuation therapy for alcohol dependence as there is a high risk of mortality if taken with alcohol.

17. A

18. B

19. C. IV diazepam should be administered ideally in a setting with access to resuscitation equipment.

20. C

21. E. Age >40 years is a risk factor for suicide.

22. C

23. B

24. D. Antidepressants should be continued for 6–9 months after the patient's mood improves.

25. C

26. D. Hyponatraemia is associated with tricyclic antidepressants, especially in the elderly population.

27. A. Venlafaxine is a drug that treats both anxiety and depression and is second-line treatment for depression after SSRIs.

28. D. Sitting sideways to the patient is less confrontational.

29. B

30. E

31. A

32. B

33. B. 10–30% of all hospital admissions are associated with alcohol.

34. C. Side-effects of lithium include hypothyroidism, hypokalaemia, raised ADH, ECG changes and renal changes.

35. A

36. C

37. C

38. E

39. C

40. E

41. E

42. A

43. B. Hyperparathyroidism and not hypoparathyroidism is a reversible cause of dementia.

44. C. Third person auditory hallucination is a positive symptom of schizophrenia.

45. A

46. E

47. A. Alternatively haloperidol 10 mg IV and diazepam 10 mg IV may be administered.

48. C

49. A. Tachycardia is a side-effect of TCAs.

50. B

51. B. In autism, imitation is impaired.

52. B

53. E

54. D

55. E

56. A. Hyperthermia and not hypothermia is associated with DTs.

57. E

58. E

59. D. Personality disorders are evident in early life.

60. B

1. A
2. D
3. G
4. F
5. O
6. D
7. K
8. A
9. E
10. G
11. C
12. D
13. F
14. G
15. J
16. C
17. B
18. F
19. I
20 H
21. I

22. C
23. B
24. L
25. F
26. A
27. G
28. K
29. J
30. M
31. A
32. C
33. L
34. F
35. H
36. C
37. D
38. A
39. G
40. F

Obstetrics and gynaecology SBAs/BOFs

In these questions candidates must select one answer only

Questions

1. In which circumstance is rhesus immunisation NOT required in a rhesus-negative mother?

   A. following amniocentesis
   B. after delivery of a rhesus-negative baby
   C. after a threatened miscarriage at 10 weeks' gestation
   D. after termination of pregnancy at 8 weeks' gestation
   E. after a spontaneous miscarriage at 12 weeks' gestation

2. Endometrial cancer is associated with all of the following EXCEPT:

   A. combined oral contraceptive pills
   B. Premarin (HRT) use in postmenopausal women with a uterus
   C. early menopause
   D. hypothyroidism
   E. multiple pregnancy

3. Routine blood tests offered at a booking antenatal clinic include all of the following EXCEPT:

   A. HIV antibody test
   B. serology for hepatitis B
   C. haemoglobin electrophoresis in a pregnant woman from India
   D. FBC
   E. clotting studies

4. Increased serum human chorionic gonadotrophin is associated with each of the following EXCEPT:

   A. choriocarcinoma
   B. hyperemesis gravidarum
   C. pregnancy
   D. ovarian carcinoma
   E. hydatidiform mole

5. Cervical smear may suggest the diagnosis of all of the following EXCEPT:

A. adenomyosis
B. bacterial vaginosis
C. *Trichomonas vaginalis*
D. CIN
E. invasive carcinoma of the cervix

6. The following statements regarding the Mirena coil are correct EXCEPT:

A. It contains levonorgestrel.
B. It controls menorrhagia.
C. It needs to be changed every 5 years.
D. It is not advisable in women with a past history of PID.
E. It increases the absolute risk of ectopic pregnancy.

7. Postcoital bleeding can occur with each of the following EXCEPT:

A. cervical polyp
B. CIN
C. *Trichomonas vaginalis* infection
D. cervical ectropion
E. endometrial carcinoma

8. Deep dyspareunia can occur with each of the following EXCEPT:

A. pelvic inflammatory disease
B. ovarian neoplasm
C. ectopic pregnancy
D. Bartholin's abscess
E. endometriosis

9. Intermenstrual bleeding may be associated with each of the following EXCEPT:

A. subserous fibroids
B. polycystic ovarian syndrome
C. carcinoma of the cervix
D. combined oral contraceptives
E. intrauterine contraceptive device

10. Appropriate investigations for a 32-year-old woman 5 days post emergency casesarean section who now presents with per vagina bleeding and passage of blood clots include all of the following EXCEPT:

   A. transvaginal ultrasound scan
   B. FBC
   C. vaginal swab for microscopy and culture
   D. LFTs
   E. clotting studies

11. Causes of preterm labour include all of the following EXCEPT:

   A. chorioamnionitis
   B. polyhydramnios
   C. cervical incompetence
   D. human papilloma virus
   E. pyelonephritis

12. Complications of pre-eclampsia include all of the following EXCEPT:

   A. IUGR
   B. renal failure
   C. thrombocytopenia
   D. cerebrovascular accident
   E. hypoglycaemia

13. A 20-year-old female is diagnosed with polycystic ovarian syndrome. She does not plan to conceive in the near future. Which treatment would you offer this patient?

   A. cyproterone acetate (Dianette)
   B. clomiphene citrate
   C. wedge resection of the ovaries
   D. Microgynon (combined oral contraceptive pill)
   E. Zoladex

14. Causes of dysmenorrhoea include all of the following EXCEPT:

   A. endometriosis
   B. IUCD (intrauterine contraceptive device)
   C. pelvic inflammatory disease
   D. subserosal fibroids
   E. polycystic ovarian disease

15. The following statements regarding ectopic pregnancy are correct EXCEPT:

    A. Risk factor includes the IUCD.
    B. It occurs in 1 in 200 pregnancies.
    C. It may present with shoulder tip pain.
    D. It never presents with bilateral lower abdominal pain.
    E. It may be treated with injection of methotrexate into the unruptured ectopic.

16. Appropriate forms of contraception after delivery for a mother who plans to breastfeed include all of the following EXCEPT:

    A. Implanon
    B. progestogen-only pill
    C. Depo-Provera
    D. IUCD
    E. combined oral contraceptive pill

17. The differential diagnosis for postmenopausal bleeding includes all of the following EXCEPT:

    A. carcinoma of the cervix
    B. adenomyosis
    C. endometrial polyp
    D. atrophic vaginitis
    E. endometrial carcinoma

18. A 14-year-old female complains of dysmenorrhoea. She states that she is not sexually active. The most appropriate medication would be:

    A. tranexamic acid
    B. mefenamic acid
    C. paracetamol
    D. Microgynon
    E. fluoxetine

19. Management of menorrhagia may include all of the following EXCEPT:

    A. norethisterone tablets 5 mg o tds for 10 days
    B. tranexamic acid 1 g o tds for 3 days
    C. placement on the combined oral contraceptive pill
    D. insertion of the Mirena intrauterine system
    E. Zoladex

20. A 20-year-old female requests emergency contraception. She had unprotected sexual intercourse 48 hours ago and has not been using any form of contraception. She has never been pregnant. Her LMP was 16 days ago. What would you offer her?

    A. combined oral contraceptive pill
    B. Levonelle-2
    C. Mirena coil
    D. Depo-Provera
    E. Implanon

21. You are summoned by the midwife to see Mrs Elliot who has just had a spontaneous vaginal delivery. She is lying in a pool of blood. The following steps in management are correct EXCEPT:

    A. Insert two large-bore venflons and take blood for FBC, clotting and T+C 2 units.
    B. Alert the obstetric registrar, senior midwife and anaesthetist.
    C. Rub the uterus and check the placenta for tears.
    D. Commence syntocinon infusion.
    E. Consent the patient for examination under anaesthesia.

22. A 50-year-old woman presents with worsening urinary incontinence over the past 2 years. She has had three SVDs and is now menopausal. She is not taking any medication. She states that the symptoms are worse when she coughs or sneezes. No prolapse is noted on pelvic examination. The following investigations are appropriate EXCEPT:

    A. urine dipstick for glucose and MSU for microscopy and culture
    B. FBC and urea/electrolytes
    C. pelvic ultrasound
    D. uroflowmetry
    E. cystometry

23. A 28-year-old obese woman presents with difficulty in conceiving. She also complains of deep pelvic pain, dysmenorrhoea and deep dyspareunia. Her cycles come every 21 days and last for 10 days. The most likely diagnosis is:

    A. polycystic ovarian disease
    B. endometriosis
    C. ovarian remnant syndrome
    D. chronic PID
    E. fibroid uterus

24. A 27-year-old woman complains of amenorrhoea for 6 months and weight gain since she quit smoking. Her UPT is negative. Her serum hormonal levels are as follows:

serum oestradiol   350 pmol/L
FSH   5 IU/L
LH   15 IU/L

The most likely diagnosis is:

A. polycystic ovarian disease
B. premature menopause
C. endometriosis
D. ovarian neoplasm
E. hydatidiform mole

25. Postcoital bleeding may be caused by each of the following EXCEPT:

A. adenomyosis
B. atrophic vaginitis
C. cervical ectropion
D. cervical polyp
E. carcinoma of the cervix

26. The most important initial investigation for a sexually active 17-year-old female complaining of lower abdominal pain and irregular vaginal bleeding is:

A. transvaginal ultrasound
B. urine pregnancy test
C. FBC
D. high vaginal and endometrial swab
E. serum βHCG and progesterone

27. Adverse effects of the combined oral contraceptive pill include all of the following EXCEPT:

A. increased risk of hepatocellular carcinoma
B. hypertension
C. a relative risk of breast cancer of 1.24
D. a three-fold increase of MI and ischaemic stroke in users with hypertension
E. a small increase in relative risk of cervical cancer with long duration of use

28. A 26-year-old woman complains of dyspareunia. On examination she is found to have a fixed, retroverted uterus and has a tender old laparotomy scar. Treatment for endometriosis may include each of the following EXCEPT:

    A. danazol
    B. norethisterone
    C. total hysterectomy with bilateral salpingo-ophorectomy
    D. diathermy
    E. clomiphene citrate

29. A 19-year-old primip. presents at 22 weeks' gestation. She is noted to have 2+ proteinuria and a BP of 170/110. She complains of frontal headache and nausea. You decide to admit her. Appropriate steps in management aside from taking blood include all of the following EXCEPT:

    A. 24-hour urine collection for protein
    B. fetal cardiotocogram
    C. consent for emergency caesarean section
    D. transabdominal ultrasound
    E. intravenous hydralazine or labetalol

30. Appropriate investigations for recurrent miscarriages include:

    A. chromosomal karyotyping of both parents
    B. screening for antiphospholipid antibody and lupus anticoagulant
    C. transvaginal ultrasound
    D. semen analysis
    E. hysterosalpingogram

Obstetrics and gynaecology EMQs
Theme: Causes of vaginal discharge

Options

A *Trichomonas vaginalis*
B Gardnerella
C Chlamydia
D Gonorrhoea
E *Mycobacterium tuberculosis*
F HIV
G Lymphogranuloma venerum
H *Treponema pallidum*
I Granuloma inguinale
J *Candida albicans*
K *Staphylococcus aureus*

For each presentation below, choose the SINGLE most likely causative organism from the above list of options. Each option may be used once, more than once, or not at all.

1. A 22-year-old woman presents with intensely irritating yellowish-green frothy vaginal discharge with severe dyspareunia. The organism is seen best under the microscope in a drop of saline.

2. A 30-year-old pregnant woman presents with a thick, white vaginal discharge associated with irritation of the vulva.

3. A 16-year-old girl who uses tampons presents with cervicitis, urethritis and unilateral Bartholin's gland inflammation.

4. A 28-year-old woman presents with acute right upper quadrant abdominal pain and watery vaginal discharge. The organism is detected by microimmunofluorescence.

5. A 23-year-old woman presents with fishy foul smelling vaginal odour. Clue cells are found in the smear.

Theme: Treatment of infertility

Options

    A Steroid suppression
    B Laparoscopy
    C Ethinyl oestradiol from days 1 to 10
    D Salpingolysis
    E Human menopausal gonadotrophins
    F Clomiphene citrate
    G Ligation of varicocoele
    H Intracytoplasmic sperm insemination
    I Artificial insemination with donor semen
    J In vitro fertilisation
    K Tubal surgery

For each case below, choose the SINGLE most appropriate treatment from the above list of options. Each option may be used once, more than once, or not at all.

6. The plasma progesterone level during the luteal phase of the cycle is absent suggesting that ovulation is not occurring. FSH and LH levels are noted to be low.

7. The cervical mucus contact test reveals agglutination of the sperm head-to-head. Sperm antibodies are also noted in the man's plasma.

8. The seminal analysis reveals severe oligospermia. The wife has patent tubes and a normal uterus.

9. The postcoital test reveals absence of sperm. The husband has a past history of mumps with orchitis. The wife has patent tubes and a normal uterus.

10. A 35-year-old woman is found to have blocked and severely diseased tubes on laparoscopy and hysterosalpingography. The uterus is normal.

Theme: Diagnosis of abdominal pain in pregnancy

Options

A Peptic ulcer disease
B Fulminating pre-eclampsia
C Appendicitis
D Abortion
E Fibroids
F Cholecystitis
G Ectopic pregnancy
H Urinary infection
I Ureteric stone
J Abruptio placentae
K Hydramnios
L Pyelonephritis

For each patient below, choose the SINGLE most likely diagnosis from the above list of options. Each option may be used once, more than once, or not at all.

11. A 33-year-old multiparous woman of 32 weeks' gestation complains of severe back pain. Urinalysis reveals red blood cells. She is apyrexial.

12. A 25-year-old primigravida of 8 weeks' gestation presents with severe lower abdominal cramping, vaginal bleeding and the passage of clots. The internal os is open.

13. A 28-year-old primigravida of 10 weeks' gestation presents with sudden, severe lower abdominal pain. The abdomen is rigid and the uterus tender.

14. A 30-year-old multiparous woman of 16 weeks' gestation presents with lower abdominal pain and tenderness. On examination she has a fundal height of 25 cm and you palpate a firm mass. She also complains of urinary frequency but denies dysuria. There is only one fetal heart beat.

15. A 26-year-old nulliparous woman of 20 weeks' gestation presents with headache and epigastric pain. BP is 150/100 and rising.

Theme: Causes of genital tract bleeding in early pregnancy

Options

A Inevitable abortion
B Missed abortion
C Complete abortion
D Threatened abortion
E Incomplete abortion
F Hydatidiform mole
G Habitual abortion
H Cervical polyp
J Cancer of the cervix
K Ectopic pregnancy
L Cervical erosion

For each case below, choose the SINGLE most likely cause from the above list of options. Each option may be used once, more than once, or not at all.

16. A nulliparous woman of 10 weeks' gestation presents with PV bleeding and pain. The internal os is open. There has been no passage of products of conception.

17. A primip. of 8 weeks' gestation presents with painless PV bleeding. Serum and urinary hCG levels are much higher than expected for her gestation.

18. A primip. of 20 weeks' gestation has a small uterus that is not consistent with her last menstrual period date. She has had no PV bleeding. She has not felt baby move all week and there are no fetal heart sounds on ultrasound.

19. A multip. of 9 weeks' gestation presents with PV bleeding. The internal os is not dilated. The cervix is normal.

20. A primip. of 10 weeks' gestation presents with PV bleeding and passage of products of conception. The cervical os remains open.

Answers to Obstetrics and gynaecology SBAs/BOFs

1. B. Guidelines for anti-D immunoglobulin suggest prophylaxis under the following sensitising circumstances: spontaneous miscarriage after 12 weeks' gestation, spontaneous miscarriage with instrumentation (TOP), threatened miscarriage at any gestation, after falls or abdominal trauma. The dose of anti-D immunoglobulin is determined according to the level of exposure to rhesus-positive blood. Anti-D should be offered within 72 hours and covers the mother for the next 6 weeks. Anti-D prophylaxis is repeated at this time if bleeding persists. Routine antenatal prophylaxis according to the Royal College of Obstetricians and Gynaecologists for all rhesus-negative women consists of two doses of at least 500 IU of anti-D immunoglobulin, the first dose at 28 weeks' gestation and the second dose at 34 weeks' gestation.

2. C. Risk factors for endometrial cancer include nulliparity, late menopause, diabetes, history of unopposed oestrogen administration, oestrogen-secreting tumours of the ovaries and obesity. Premarin is a form of unopposed oestrogen HRT and should only be administered to women post hysterectomy.

3. E. Routine blood tests offered at booking clinic include full blood count, blood group and antibody screen, serology for hepatitis B (not A!), syphilis, rubella and HIV. Sickle-cell test and haemoglobin electrophoresis are also offered to at-risk patients.

4. D. Increased levels of human chorionic gonadotrophin have been associated with choriocarcinoma, hyperemesis gravidarum, pregnancy and hydatidiform mole. Hepatoma may be associated with increased levels of alpha-fetoprotein. Ovarian cancer may be associated with elevated CA-125.

5. A. Cervical smear may pick up incidental infections such as *Trichomonas vaginalis*, bacterial vaginosis (gardnerella), actinomyces and candida. Cervical smear may reveal mild to severe dysplasia which is suggestive of low to high grade CIN. Severe dyskaryosis with additional features may suggest invasive carcinoma. Dyskaryotic glandular cells may

represent adenocarcinoma of the endometrium or endocervical adenocarcinoma in situ.

6. E. The Mirena coil or the levonorgestrel-releasing intrauterine system (IUS) is licensed to be used for 5 years at a time in the UK. It does not have a product licence yet for control of menorrhagia but it does have this added advantage. The local effect of the Mirena coil causes thickening of the cervical mucus, endometrial atrophy and partial ovulation suppression. It is not advisable in patients with a past history of PID and does not increase the risk of ectopic pregnancy. By acting as a contraceptive device with 99% efficacy, the risk is lower.

7. E. Postcoital bleeding is associated with cervical polyp, cervical ectropion, carcinoma of the cervix, infection with *Trichomonas vaginalis*, which may appear as a strawberry cervix, and atrophic vaginitis.

8. D. Deep dyspareunia is associated with PID, endometriosis, ectopic pregnancy, ovarian neoplasm and chronic pelvic pain. Superficial dyspareunia is associated with vulvar, vaginal or urethral pathology.

9. A. Intermenstrual bleeding may be associated with infection in patients with a IUCD in situ and with intramural or submucous fibroids.

10. D. The differential diagnosis in this situation includes endometritis, retained products of conception, haematoma and breakdown of sutures.

11. D. Other causes for preterm labour include procedures such as amniocentesis, multiple pregnancy and an abnormal uterus.

12. E. Other potential complications of pre-eclampsia include fits, disseminated intracellular coagulopathy (DIC) and maternal death.

13. A. Dianette oral contraceptive pill contains the antiandrogen cytoproterone acetate.

14. D. Causes of dysmenorrhoea include endometriosis, misplaced IUCD, pelvic inflammatory disease, ovarian tumour, history of sexual abuse, and prior abdominal or pelvic surgery. Fibroids are associated with menorrhagia. PCO are associated with amenorrhoea.

15. D. An ectopic pregnancy is a pregnancy that occurs outside the uterine cavity. The majority occurs in the fallopian tube. Isthmial pregnancies may rupture between 4 and 8 weeks as the wall of the medial two-thirds of the tube cannot stretch. Ampullary pregnancies may rupture between 8 and 12 weeks, as the muscle wall of the lateral one-third of the tube is lax. It occurs in 1 in 200 pregnancies and is associated with salpingitis, tubal surgery, IUCD, etc. It may present with shoulder tip pain due to diaphragmatic irritation from accumulated blood. The abdominal pain may be bilateral or unilateral. Classically, the patient will have sudden severe lower quadrant abdominal pain, a rigid abdomen, a very tender uterus and a boggy adnexal mass.

16. E. The combined oral contraceptive pill contains oestrogen, which is absorbed in breast milk and therefore should not be offered as postpartum contraception.

17. B. The differential diagnosis for postmenopausal bleeding includes carcinoma of the cervix and endometrium, endometrial polyp and atrophic vaginitis. A speculum examination of the cervix and cervical smear are indicated. An urgent transvaginal ultrasound should be arranged to assess for endometrial hyperplasia or the presence of a polyp. A pipelle biopsy of the endometrium can then be taken if the endometrium is thickened.

18. B

19. E

20. A. Emergency contraception in the form of Levonelle-2 may be offered up to 72 hours after unprotected sexual intercourse. The IUCD may be offered up to 5 days post unprotected sexual intercourse. The Mirena coil is not recommended for emergency contraception.

21. A. The patient should be typed and crossed for 6 units of blood!

22. B

23. B

24. A. PCO is associated with a serum LH/FSH ratio of 3. Diagnosis is confirmed by transvaginal ultrasound that will demonstrate the typical follicles surrounding the ovary.

25. A. Postcoital bleeding may be caused by atrophic vaginitis, cervical ectropion, cervical carcinoma, or cervical polyp. Cervical ectropion is eversion of the lower cervical canal and is associated with the 3 'p's' – puberty, pregnancy and the combined oral contraceptive pill. It is usually asymptomatic but can present with postcoital bleeding. Treatment involves cryotherapy.

26. B. The diagnosis of ectopic pregnancy should be excluded.

27. B

28. E

29. C

30. D

Answers to Obstetrics and gynaecology EMQs

1. A
2. J
3. D
4. C
5. B
6. F
7. A
8. H
9. I
10. J
11. I
12. D
13. G
14. E
15. B
16. A
17. F
18. B
19. D
20. E

In these questions candidates must select one answer only

Questions

1. A 7-year-old boy presents with an itchy anus. His mother states that the itching is worse at night in bed. The most likely diagnosis is:

   A. enterobiasis
   B. ascariasis
   C. scabies
   D. body lice
   E. crab lice

2. Treatment for this boy would be:

   A. Derbac-M
   B. malathion
   C. mebendazole
   D. pyrantel pamoate
   E. permethrin

3. A 10-year-old boy presents with allergic nasal polyps. What is the best treatment for this boy?

   A. Betnesol nasal drops
   B. Clarityn
   C. Zirtek
   D. saline nasal drops
   E. xylometazoline nasal drops

4. A 4-year-old boy presents with fever, epistaxis and pain in his legs. On examination he has hepatosplenomegaly. The most useful blood test is:

   A. LFTs
   B. FBC
   C. urea/electrolytes
   D. ESR
   E. creatinine kinase

5. A 15-year-old girl presents with fever and sore throat. On examination there is an exudate over both tonsils. She has no drug allergies. The most appropriate treatment is:

   A. amoxicillin
   B. penicillin
   C. metronidazole
   D. ciprofloxacin
   E. co-amoxiclavulanic acid

6. A 5-year-old boy presents with a maculopapular rash on his buttocks and ankles. He also complains of abdominal pain and knee pain. The most likely diagnosis is:

   A. rheumatic fever
   B. juvenile chronic arthritis
   C. coeliac disease
   D. Henoch–Schönlein syndrome
   E. chickenpox

7. A 4-year-old girl presents with pallor, irritability, abdominal distension and fatty diarrhoea. Full blood count shows both a macrocytic and microcytic anaemia. The next most useful investigation is:

   A. sweat sodium and chloride test
   B. abdominal x-ray
   C. hydrogen breath test
   D. endomysial antibody
   E. abdominal ultrasound

8. A 6-week-old baby boy is brought in by his mother for failure to thrive. He vomits his food across the room after each feed. His mother states that he is always hungry. The most useful investigation is:

   A. test feed
   B. contrast enema
   C. ultrasound
   D. abdominal x-ray
   E. sweat chloride test

9. Treatment would be:

    A. oral rehydration therapy
    B. Ramstedt's operation
    C. reduction with contrast enema
    D. gluten-free diet
    E. pancreatic enzyme supplementation

10. An 18-month-old baby presents with fever and vomiting. The throat, chest and abdomen are normal on examination. The most likely diagnosis is:

    A. gastroenteritis
    B. viral meningitis
    C. pharyngeal pouch
    D. intussusception
    E. congenital hiatal hernia

11. An 8-year-old girl presents with fever, drowsiness and a non-blanching rash. The most likely diagnosis is:

    A. infectious mononucleosis
    B. meningitis
    C. scarlet fever
    D. chickenpox
    E. Kawasaki's syndrome

12. The most useful investigation is:

    A. FBC
    B. blood cultures
    C. lumbar puncture
    D. monospot test
    E. throat swab

13. The most appropriate treatment is:

    A. benzylpenicillin
    B. erythromycin
    C. aspirin
    D. chloramphenicol
    E. cefuroxime

14. A 3-month-old baby is brought in by her mother. She explains that the baby has frequent screaming spells. The baby is being bottle-fed. The most appropriate treatment for colic would be:

A. change formula to soya milk
B. give sugar water
C. add karo syrup to formula
D. peppermint oil
E. mebeverine

15. An 18-month-old boy presents with fever, bleeding from the lips and an erythematous rash over the face and trunk. The boy does not like to hold anything in his hands and refuses to stand up. The most likely diagnosis is:

A. streptococcal scarlet fever
B. leptospirosis
C. Epstein–Barr viral infection
D. erythema multiforme
E. Kawasaki's syndrome

16. The most appropriate management would be:

A. admit the boy to hospital and give daily aspirin
B. admit the boy to hospital for IV penicillin
C. admit the boy to hospital for IV corticosteroids
D. treat as an outpatient with oral penicillin
E. treat at home symptomatically with Calpol (paracetamol) prn

17. A 4-month-old baby is brought in by his mother. She states that he had been coughing for a few days and is now wheezing and breathless. On examination the baby is febrile with a temperature of 38°C and is breathing at a rate of 70 per minute with intercostal recession. Widespread rales and rhonchi are present on auscultation of the chest. The most likely diagnosis is:

A. asthma
B. pneumonia
C. bronchiolitis
D. whooping cough
E. acute laryngotracheitis

18. A 7-year-old boy presents with fever, vomiting and abdominal pain. On examination he is tender in the periumbilical region and in the right lower abdomen. He looks pale and has no appetite. The most likely diagnosis is:

A. intussusception
B. gastroenteritis
C. cystic fibrosis
D. appendicitis
E. ulcerative colitis

19. A 14-year-old girl presents with vomiting and severe abdominal pain. She states that she had a sore throat a week ago. This afternoon, she had been playing rugby at school and been knocked in her side. On examination she is pale, apyrexial and acutely tender in the left upper abdomen. The most likely diagnosis is:

A. splenic rupture
B. hepatic rupture
C. acute appendicitis
D. perforated peptic ulcer
E. acute intestinal obstruction

20. For which condition is the pneumococcal vaccine indicated over the age of 2?

A. cerebral palsy
B. coeliac disease
C. sickle-cell trait
D. diabetes insipidus
E. cystic fibrosis

21. A 4-year-old girl is brought in by her mother. The mother states that her daughter is suffering from nightmares and snores. She has a history of recurrent ear infections. On examination the child has large tonsils and has nasal speech. The most likely diagnosis is:

A. adenoidal hyperplasia
B. sleep apnoea
C. asthma
D. nasal polyps
E. gastro-oesophageal reflux disease

22. A 12-year-old girl presents with a pink macular truncal rash and suboccipital lymphadenopathy. The most likely diagnosis is:

A. mumps
B. chickenpox
C. rubella
D. measles
E. erythema infectiosum

23. A 10-month-old baby presents with high fever and catarrh for 3 days. This is followed by a light red, macular rash over her trunk. The mother states that the baby is improving. The most likely diagnosis is:

A. erythema infectiosum
B. rubella
C. roseola infantum
D. Kawasaki's syndrome
E. measles

24. A 6-year-old girl presents with fever and vesicles on the palms and soles and in the mouth. She is drooling saliva and is very irritable. The most likely aetiology is:

A. coxsackie A16 virus infection
B. herpes simplex virus infection
C. human parvovirus type B12
D. *Trepenoma pallidum*
E. measles

25. A 15-year-old presents with an oval pink rash. She states that it started with a single patch that became scaly but has now spread all over her chest. The most likely diagnosis is:

A. scarlet fever
B. pityriasis rosea
C. rubella
D. psoriasis
E. discoid eczema

26. A 6-month-old baby is brought in with a nappy rash. On examination the rash is isolated red plaques and covered with silvery scales. The most likely diagnosis is:

A. ammonia dermatitis
B. seborrhoeic eczema dermatitis
C. candida dermatitis
D. psoriatic dermatitis
E. cellulitis

27. The following are recognised causes of short stature EXCEPT for:

A. achondroplasia
B. coeliac disease
C. hypopituitarism
D. homocystinuria
E. constitutional

28. An 8-year-old girl presents with epistaxis and knee pain. On examination she is pale, tachycardic and apyrexial. A pan-systolic murmur is auscultated. She has a serpiginous red, raised rash over her trunk and non-tender subcutaneous nodules near her joints. The most likely diagnosis is:

A. idiopathic thrombocytopenic purpura
B. juvenile rheumatoid arthritis
C. Kawasaki's disease
D. rubella
E. rheumatic fever

29. The following investigations are indicated EXCEPT:

A. 12-lead ECG
B. FBC
C. ESR
D. antistreptolysin O test
E. creatinine kinase

30. The most appropriate treatment is:

A. aspirin
B. benzylpenicillin
C. corticosteroid therapy
D. NSAIDs
E. cefuroxime

Paediatric EMQs
Theme: Diagnosis of childhood illnesses

Option

A Measles
B Rubella
C Varicella zoster
D Mumps
E Erythema infectiosum
F Infectious mononucleosis
G Tuberculosis
H Typhus
I Kawasaki's syndrome
J Pneumococcal meningitis
K *Haemophilus influenzae* epiglottitis
L Streptococcal throat infection

For each patient below, choose the SINGLE most likely diagnosis from the above list of options. Each option may be used once, more than once, or not at all.

1. A 15-year-old girl presents with fever, cough, coryza and conjunctivitis 9 days after exposure. On examination, she has blue-white punctate lesions on the buccal mucosa.

2. A 17-year-old boy presents with fever, stridor and trismus. He is noted to be drooling saliva. On examination he has palpable neck nodes. He fails to respond to a course of penicillin.

3. A 7-year-old girl presents with a low grade fever and a 'slapped cheek', erythematous eruption on her cheeks.

4. A 4-year-old boy presents with an acute onset of fever and a vesicular eruption, following an incubation period of 12 days. The vesicles evolve into pustules and crust over.

5. A 1-year-old baby boy presents with a 5-day history of fever, strawberry tongue, and erythema of the palms and soles. He also has an enlarged 2 cm lymph node.

Theme: Investigation of failure to thrive

Options

    A FBC
    B Sweat test
    C Urinalysis
    D Serum electrolytes
    E Bone films
    F TFTs
    G Buccal smear (females)
    H Stool culture
    I Echocardiogram
    J Fasting blood glucose
    K Abdominal ultrasound

For each presentation below, choose the SINGLE most discriminating investigation from the above list of options. Each option may be used once, more than once, or not at all.

6.   A small 6-year-old boy on regular salbutamol inhaler presents with nasal obstruction and persistent cough. On examination he is found to have nasal polyps.

7.   A 2-year-old boy presents with anorexia, impaired growth, abdominal distension, abnormal stools and hypotonia. He is irritable when examined.

8.   A 14-year-old girl presents with anorexia. She reports that her appetite is good but cannot seem to gain weight. Her parents describe her as hyperactive and emotional. Blood pressure is 130/80 and pulse rate 108/min.

9.   A 5-year-old boy presents with weight loss and nocturnal enuresis. His parents describe him as having profound mood swings. They have attempted to limit his fluid intake at night.

10. A 6-week-old baby presents with failure to thrive. The mother reports that he takes 1 hour for feeding with frequent rests. On examination he is tachycardic, tachypnoeic and has an enlarged liver.

Theme: Investigations of paediatric emergencies

Options

    A FBC
    B Serum glucose
    C Skull x-ray
    D Chest x-ray
    E Urinalysis
    F ESR
    G Serum urea and electrolytes
    H CT scan of the head
    I Lateral soft-tissue neck x-ray

For each case below, choose the SINGLE most discriminating investigation from the above list of options. Each option may be used once, more than once, or not at all.

11. An 8-month-old baby is brought to Casualty by her mother after falling off the sofa on to her head. On examination she is irritable and alert, with no lateralising signs. There is a haematoma over her left occiput.

12. A 6-year-old girl is brought to Casualty by her mother after falling off a climbing frame in the school playground. On examination there is no deformity or swelling of her extremities. Instead she has bruising of various colours over her arms and tender ribs on palpation.

13. A 2-year-old girl is brought to Casualty by her father after falling down the stairs. She is drowsy and has vomited twice. On examination there is a swelling over her occiput. Her pupils are sluggish to respond. Blood pressure is 120/70 and pulse rate is 60.

14. A 2-year-old boy has swallowed a 50 pence coin and points to his throat. He is not distressed.

15. A 4-year-old girl is brought to Casualty with severe left shoulder and left upper abdominal pain. Temperature is 40°C. Breath sounds are decreased in the left lung base. Urine dipstick shows scant red blood cells.

Theme: Management of paediatric gastrointestinal disorders

Options

    A Vancomycin
    B Panproctocolectomy
    C Gluten-free diet
    D Pancreatic enzyme supplementation
    E Barium enema
    F Rectal biopsy
    G D-penicillamine and avoidance of chocolates, nuts and shellfish
    H Diverting colostomy
    I Loperamide

For each case below, choose the SINGLE most appropriate management option from the above list of options. Each option may be used once, more than once, or not at all.

16. A 2-year-old girl presents with failure to thrive and diarrhoea. She is found to have iron-deficiency anaemia. Small bowel biopsy shows flattened villi, elongated crypts and loss of columnar cells.

17. A 12-year-old boy is being treated for osteomyelitis. He has been on intravenous antibiotics for 2 weeks. He now has diarrhoea. On sigmoidoscopy there are multiple patchy yellowish areas of necrotic mucosa.

18. A 6-month-old baby boy presents with repeated bouts of vomiting and abdominal distension. He is normal between attacks. A sausage-shaped mass is palpated in his abdomen.

19. A 2-month-old baby girl presents with failure to thrive. She has frequent episodes of vomiting with abdominal distension. Abdominal x-ray shows proximal bowel dilatation and no faeces or gas in the rectum.

20. A 12-year-old boy presents with liver disease. A slit-lamp examination reveals Kayser–Fleischer rings in his cornea. Urinary copper level is high.

Answers to Paediatric SBAs/BOFs

1. A

2. C

3. A

4. B. The diagnosis is most likely acute lymphoblastic leukaemia.

5. B. The patient may have glandular fever, which can be confirmed by monospot test. If a strep. throat, is suspected, give penicillin. Amoxicillin should never be prescribed for sore throat as the patient may have infectious mononucleosis and develop a drug rash to amoxicillin as well as classically to ampicillin.

6. D

7. D. Endomysial antibody suggests coeliac disease. Definitive diagnosis is made by jejunal biopsy.

8. A. On test feed, an olive-shaped mass may be palpated and visible peristalsis evident in pyloric stenosis.

9. B

10. A

11. B

12. C

13. A

14. A

15. E. The boy will refuse his toys and refuse to stand as the palms and soles will be red and indurated.

16. A. There is a risk of coronary artery aneurysm associated with Kawasaki's disease.

17. C

18. D. Periumbilical pain then shifts to the McBurney's point in appendicitis.

19. A. The girl most likely had infectious mononucleosis, which carries a risk of splenic rupture and contact sports should be avoided for up to 6 weeks post infection.

20. B. Other conditions include diabetes mellitus, sickle-cell anaemia and asplenia.

21. A. Adenoidal hyperplasia may present with night terrors, an adenoid facies, Eustachian tube dysfunction and snoring. ENT referral should be made for PNS examination.

22. C

23. A. The disease is self-limiting.

24. A. This child has hand, foot and mouth disease.

25. B. Pityriasis rosea is a self-limiting viral illness associated with a Herald's patch.

26. D

27. D. Homocystinuria is associated with tall stature.

28. E. Fever is not always present in cases of acute rheumatic fever so do not be misled.

29. E

30. B

Answers to Paediatric EMQs

1. A. Koplik spots are seen prior to the measles rash.

2. F. This is a patient with glandular fever and upper airway obstruction.

3. E

4. C

5. I

6. B. Cystic fibrosis is diagnosed by an abnormally high sweat chloride level.

7. A. Coeliac disease is suggested by a mixed anaemia (iron and folic acid deficiencies). However the definitive diagnosis is made by diagnosis of the jejunum.

8. F. This is a case of hyperthyroidism.

9. J. This is a case of juvenile-onset diabetes mellitus.

10. I. The four classic signs of congestive heart failure include tachycardia, tachypnoea, cardiomegaly and hepatomegaly.

11. C. A CT scan of the head is unnecessary in the absence of signs of increased intracranial pressure. A skull x-ray to look for skull fracture is more than adequate.

12. D. Non-accidental injury should be considered here. A chest x-ray to exclude rib fractures is required.

13. H. This child is experiencing signs of increased intra-cranial pressure with hypertension and bradycardia. For a 2-year-old, the resting heart rate should be greater than 95 beats/min. The blood pressure is too high for a 2-year-old.

14. D. In a 2-year-old, an AP chest view will more than adequately image the neck and chest to reveal a radio-opaque coin lodged in the cricopharyngeal region.

15. D. This 4-year-old should be investigated for left basal pneumonia. She clearly has diaphragmatic irritation. The edge of the kidney is being irritated leading to leakage of red blood cells. This is an actual patient case!

16. C. The patient has coeliac disease.

17. A. The patient has developed pseudomembranous colitis, which is treated with vancomycin or metronidazole.

18. E. The baby has intussusception. This can be both diagnosed and treated by barium enema. However mortality is still 1% due to a delay in diagnosis and treatment.

19. F. This baby may have Hirschsprung's disease, which is confirmed by rectal biopsy.

20. G. This patient most likely has Wilson's disease and should avoid copper-containing foods.